Nutrition in Older Adults

Editor

JOHN E. MORLEY

CLINICS IN
GERIATRIC MEDICINE

www.geriatric.theclinics.com

August 2015 • Volume 31 • Number 3

ELSEVIER

1600 John F. Kennedy Boulevard • Suite 1800 • Philadelphia, Pennsylvania, 19103-2899

http://www.theclinics.com

CLINICS IN GERIATRIC MEDICINE Volume 31, Number 3
August 2015 ISSN 0749–0690, ISBN-13: 978-0-323-41332-9

Editor: Jessica McCool
Developmental Editor: Colleen Viola

Clinics in Geriatric Medicine (ISSN 0749-0690) is published quarterly by Elsevier Inc., 360 Park Avenue South, New York, NY 10010-1710. Months of issue are February, May, August, and November. Business and Editorial Offices: 1600 John F. Kennedy Blvd., Suite 1800, Philadelphia, PA 191023-2899. Periodicals postage paid at New York, NY, and additional mailing offices. Subscription prices are $280.00 per year (US individuals), $498.00 per year (US institutions), $145.00 per year (US student/resident), $370.00 per year (Canadian individuals), $632.00 per year (Canadian institutions), $195.00 per year (Canadian student/resident), $390.00 per year (international individuals), $632.00 per year (international institutions), and $195.00 per year (international student/resident). Foreign air speed delivery is included in all *Clinics* subscription prices. All prices are subject to change without notice. POSTMASTER: Send address changes to *Clinics in Geriatric Medicine,* Elsevier Health Sciences Division, Subscription Customer Service, 3251 Riverport Lane, Maryland Heights, MO 63043. **Telephone: 1-800-654-2452 (U.S. and Canada); 314-447-8871 (outside U.S. and Canada). Fax: 314-447-8029. E-mail:** journalscustomerservice-usa@elsevier.com **(for print support) or** journalsonlinesupport-usa@elsevier.com **(for online support).**

Reprints. For copies of 100 or more, of articles in this publication, please contact the Commercial Reprints Department, Elsevier Inc., 360 Park Avenue South, New York, New York 10010-1710. Tel.: 212-633-3874; Fax: 212-633-3820, E-mail: reprints@elsevier.com.

Clinics in Geriatric Medicine is covered in *MEDLINE/PubMed (Index Medicus), EMBASE/Excerpta Medica, Current Contents/Clinical Medicine (CC/CM), and the Cumulative Index to Nursing & Allied Health Literature.*

Contributors

EDITOR

JOHN E. MORLEY, MB, BCh
Dammert Professor of Medicine and Director, Division of Geriatric Medicine; Division of Endocrinology, Saint Louis University School of Medicine, St Louis, Missouri

AUTHORS

AHMED H. ABDELHAFIZ, MSc, MD, FRCP
Consultant Physician and Honorary Senior Clinical Lecturer, Department of Elderly Medicine, Rotherham General Hospital, Rotherham, United Kingdom

SANDRINE ANDRIEU, MD, PhD
INSERM UMR 1027; University of Toulouse III; Department of Epidemiology and Public Health, CHU Toulouse, Toulouse, France

RITA DE CÁSSIA AQUINO, PhD
Nutrition Department, São Judas Tadeu University, São Paulo, Brazil

CONNIE W. BALES, PhD, RD
Department of Medicine, Duke University Medical Center; Durham VA Medical Center, Geriatric Research, Education and Clinical Center, Durham, North Carolina

JUERGEN M. BAUER, MD, PhD
Department of Geriatric Medicine, Carl von Ossietzky Universität Oldenburg, Klinikum Oldenburg gGmbH, Oldenburg, Germany

ROBERTO BERNABEI, MD
Department of Geriatrics, Neurosciences and Orthopedics, Catholic University of the Sacred Heart, Rome, Italy

RICCARDO CALVANI, PhD
Department of Geriatrics, Neurosciences and Orthopedics, Catholic University of the Sacred Heart, Rome, Italy

TOMMY CEDERHOLM, MD
Professor of Clinical Nutrition; Senior Consultant in Geriatric Medicine, Department of Public Health and Caring Sciences, Clinical Nutrition and Metabolism, Uppsala University, Uppsala, Sweden

MATTEO CESARI, MD, PhD
Gérontopôle, University Hospital of Toulouse, Toulouse, France

NICOLA COLEY, PhD
INSERM UMR 1027; University of Toulouse III; Department of Epidemiology and Public Health, CHU Toulouse, Toulouse, France

ALFONSO J. CRUZ-JENTOFT, MD
Head of the Geriatric Department, University Hospital Ramón y Cajal, Madrid, Spain

REBECCA DIEKMANN, PhD
Department of Geriatric Medicine, Carl von Ossietzky Universität Oldenburg, Klinikum Oldenburg gGmbH, Oldenburg, Germany

SOPHIE GUYONNET, PhD
Gérontopôle, Toulouse University Hospital; INSERM UMR 1027; Toulouse III Paul Sabatier University, Toulouse, France

MICHAEL HOROWITZ, MBBS, PhD, FRACP
Discipline of Medicine, National Health and Medical Research Council of Australia (NHMRC) Centre of Research Excellence in Translating Nutritional Science to Good Health, Royal Adelaide Hospital, The University of Adelaide, Adelaide, South Australia, Australia

KAREN L. JONES, Dip App Sci, PhD
Discipline of Medicine, National Health and Medical Research Council of Australia (NHMRC) Centre of Research Excellence in Translating Nutritional Science to Good Health, Royal Adelaide Hospital, The University of Adelaide, Adelaide, South Australia, Australia

SEEMA JOSHI, MD
Medical Director, Community Living Center, Department of Geriatrics and Extended Care, Veterans Affairs Medical Center, Leavenworth, Kansas; Assistant Professor, Division of Health Services Research, Department of Internal Medicine, University of Kansas Medical Center, Kansas City, Kansas

FRANCESCO LANDI, MD, PhD
Department of Geriatrics, Neurosciences and Orthopedics, Catholic University of the Sacred Heart, Rome, Italy

SILMARA DOS SANTOS LUZ, PhD
Research Group of Nutrition, Physical Activity and Aging Processes, University of São Paulo, São Paulo, Brazil

ANNA MARIA MARTONE, MD
Department of Geriatrics, Neurosciences and Orthopedics, Catholic University of the Sacred Heart, Rome, Italy

EMANUELE MARZETTI, MD, PhD
Department of Geriatrics, Neurosciences and Orthopedics, Catholic University of the Sacred Heart, Rome, Italy

JEAN-PIERRE MICHEL, MD
Emeritus Professor of Medicine, Geneva University, Geneva, Switzerland

JOHN E. MORLEY, MB, BCh
Dammert Professor of Medicine and Director, Division of Geriatric Medicine; Division of Endocrinology, Saint Louis University School of Medicine, St Louis, Missouri

GRAZIANO ONDER, MD, PhD
Department of Geriatrics, Neurosciences and Orthopedics, Catholic University of the Sacred Heart, Rome, Italy

KATHRYN N. PORTER STARR, PhD, RD
Department of Medicine, Duke University Medical Center; Durham VA Medical Center, Geriatric Research, Education and Clinical Center, Durham, North Carolina

CHRIS K. RAYNER, MBBS, PhD, FRACP
Discipline of Medicine, National Health and Medical Research Council of Australia (NHMRC) Centre of Research Excellence in Translating Nutritional Science to Good Health, Royal Adelaide Hospital, The University of Adelaide, Adelaide, South Australia, Australia

SANDRA MARIA LIMA RIBEIRO, PhD
Research Group of Nutrition, Physical Activity and Aging Processes, Department of Gerontology, University of São Paulo, São Paulo, Brazil

YVES ROLLAND, MD, PhD
Gérontopôle, Toulouse University Hospital; INSERM UMR 1027; Toulouse III Paul Sabatier University, Toulouse, France

ALAN J. SINCLAIR, MSc, MD, FRCP
Professor of Medicine, Foundation for Diabetes Research in Older People, Diabetes Frail Ltd, Droitwich Spa, United Kingdom

STIJN SOENEN, PhD
Discipline of Medicine, National Health and Medical Research Council of Australia (NHMRC) Centre of Research Excellence in Translating Nutritional Science to Good Health, Royal Adelaide Hospital, The University of Adelaide, Adelaide, South Australia, Australia

MATTEO TOSATO, MD, PhD
Department of Geriatrics, Neurosciences and Orthopedics, Catholic University of the Sacred Heart, Rome, Italy

CHARLOTTE VAURS, MD
INSERM UMR 1027; University of Toulouse III; Nutrition Unit, Department of Endocrinology, CHU Toulouse, Toulouse, France

RENUKA VISVANATHAN, MBBS, FRACP, PhD
Professor (Geriatric Medicine); Clinical Director, Aged and Extended Care Services, The Queen Elizabeth Hospital, Central Adelaide Local Health Network; Director, Adelaide Geriatrics Training and Research with Aged Care (GTRAC) Centre, School of Medicine, University of Adelaide, Adelaide, South Australia, Australia

Contents

Preface: Novel Approaches to Nutrition in Older Persons **xiii**

John E. Morley

Excessive Body Weight in Older Adults **311**

Kathryn N. Porter Starr and Connie W. Bales

The health challenges prompted by obesity in the older adult population are poorly recognized and understudied. A defined treatment of geriatric obesity is difficult to establish, as it must take into account biological heterogeneity, age-related comorbidities, and functional limitations (sarcopenia/dynapenia). This retrospective article highlights the current understanding of the optimal body mass index (BMI) in later life, addressing appropriate recommendations based on BMI category, age, and health history. The findings of randomized control trials of weight loss/maintenance interventions help one to move closer to evidence-based and appropriately individualized recommendations for body weight management in older adults.

Protein and Older Persons **327**

Juergen M. Bauer and Rebecca Diekmann

An optimal protein intake is important for the preservation of muscle mass, functionality, and quality of life in older persons. In recent years, new recommendations regarding the optimal intake of protein in this population have been published. Based on the available scientific literature, 1.0 to 1.2 g protein/kg body weight (BW)/d are recommended in healthy older adults. In certain disease states, a daily protein intake of more than 1.2 g/kg BW may be required. The distribution of protein intake over the day, the amount per meal, and the amino acid profile of proteins are also discussed.

Gastric Emptying in the Elderly **339**

Stijn Soenen, Chris K. Rayner, Michael Horowitz, and Karen L. Jones

Aging is characterized by a diminished homeostatic regulation of physiologic functions, including slowing of gastric emptying. Gastric and small intestinal motor and humoral mechanisms in humans are complex and highly variable: ingested food is stored, mixed with digestive enzymes, ground into small particles, and delivered as a liquefied form into the duodenum at a rate allowing efficient digestion and absorption. In healthy aging, motor function is well preserved whereas deficits in sensory function are more apparent. The effects of aging on gastric emptying are relevant to the absorption of oral medications and the regulation of appetite, postprandial glycemia, and blood pressure.

Vitamin Supplementation in the Elderly **355**

Seema Joshi

Vitamin supplementation is fairly common among the elderly. Supplements are often used to prevent disease and improve health. In the

United States, the use of dietary supplements has continued to increase over the last 30 years, and more than half of adults report using one or more dietary supplements. Epidemiologic evidence suggests that a diet rich in fruits and vegetables does have a protective effect on health. However, clinical trials on the use of vitamin supplements for promotion of health and prevention of disease have failed to demonstrate the strong associations seen in observational studies.

Sarcopenia as the Biological Substrate of Physical Frailty **367**

Francesco Landi, Riccardo Calvani, Matteo Cesari, Matteo Tosato, Anna Maria Martone, Roberto Bernabei, Graziano Onder, and Emanuele Marzetti

Physical function decreases with aging, which may result in adverse outcomes (eg, disability, loss of independence, institutionalization, death). Physical function impairment is a common trait of frailty and sarcopenia. These two conditions, albeit highly common, have not yet received a unique operational definition, which has impeded their implementation in standard practice. Here, we introduce a conceptual model in which sarcopenia is proposed as the biological substrate and the pathway whereby the consequences of physical frailty develop. This conceptualization may open new venues for the design of interventions against physical frailty and promote the translation of findings to the clinical arena.

Frailty, Exercise and Nutrition **375**

Jean-Pierre Michel, Alfonso J. Cruz-Jentoft, and Tommy Cederholm

This article first reports the spontaneous course of frailty conditions, and then focuses on randomized, controlled frailty interventions (such as physical exercise, nutrition, combined exercise plus nutrition, and multifactorial interventions) or metaanalysis in community-dwelling older adults or volunteers published in 2012, 2013, and 2014. The main take-home messages that emerge from recent literature are summarized.

Dehydration, Hypernatremia, and Hyponatremia **389**

John E. Morley

Disturbances of serum sodium are one of the most common findings in older persons. They are also a major cause of hospital admissions and delirium and are associated with frailty, falls, and hip fractures. Both hypernatremia and hyponatremia are potentially preventable. Treatment involves treating the underlying cause and restoring sodium and volume status to normal. The arginine vasopressin antagonists, vaptans, have increased the therapeutic armamentarium available to physicians.

The Role of Nutrition and Physical Activity in Cholesterol and Aging **401**

Sandra Maria Lima Ribeiro, Silmara dos Santos Luz, and Rita de Cássia Aquino

Cholesterol is a precursor of several substances with important biologic activities; however, it is common to associate this molecule only with bad outcomes. This article reviews the cholesterol metabolism, its functions in the human body, its pathogenicity, and its elimination. The modifications in biochemical paths of cholesterol in aging are highlighted. Finally, the role of diet, physical activity, and exercise in cholesterol management is discussed.

Anorexia of Aging **417**

Renuka Visvanathan

The anorexia of aging is common, leading to adverse health consequences. As populations age, the impacts from anorexia in the older population are set to increase. Only greater awareness will allow for prevention or early intervention. This article discusses the physiologic anorexia of aging, highlights contributing factors, and proposes management strategies, including screening, especially in primary care. Many neuroendocrine factors have been implicated in the pathophysiology; it is clear that further human research is necessary if there is to be a pharmacologic breakthrough. There are currently no approved pharmacologic treatment strategies to prevent or treat the anorexia of aging.

Screening for Malnutrition in Older People **429**

Sophie Guyonnet and Yves Rolland

Malnutrition risk increases with age and level of care. Despite significant medical advances, malnutrition remains a significant and highly prevalent public health problem of developed countries. Earlier identification and appropriate nutrition support may help to reverse or halt the malnutrition trajectory and the negative outcomes associated with poor nutritional status. A nutrition screening process is recommended to help detect people with protein-energy malnutrition (PEM) or at malnutrition risk. Evidence supports that oral nutritional supplements and dietary counseling can increase dietary intake and improve quality of life in elderly with PEM or at malnutrition risk. This article examines nutritional screening and assessment tools designated for older adults.

Diabetes, Nutrition, and Exercise **439**

Ahmed H. Abdelhafiz and Alan J. Sinclair

Aging is associated with body composition changes that lead to glucose intolerance and increased risk of diabetes. The incidence of diabetes increases with aging, and the prevalence has increased because of the increased life expectancy of the population. Lifestyle modifications through nutrition and exercise in combination with medications are the main components of diabetes management. The potential benefits of nutrition and exercise intervention in older people with diabetes are enormous. Nutrition and exercise training are feasible even in frail older people living in care homes and should take into consideration individual circumstances, cultural factors, and ethnic preferences.

Nutrition and Cognition in Aging Adults **453**

Nicola Coley, Charlotte Vaurs, and Sandrine Andrieu

Numerous longitudinal observational studies have suggested that nutrients, such as antioxidants, B vitamins, and ω-3 fatty acids, may prevent cognitive decline or dementia. There is very little evidence from well-sized randomized controlled trials that nutritional interventions can benefit cognition in later life. Nutritional interventions may be more effective in individuals with poorer nutritional status or as part of multidomain interventions simultaneously targeting multiple lifestyle factors. Further evidence, notably from randomized controlled trials, is required to prove or refute these hypotheses.

Index **465**

CLINICS IN GERIATRIC MEDICINE

FORTHCOMING ISSUES

November 2015
Geriatric Urology
Tomas L. Griebling, *Editor*

February 2016
Geriatric Oncology
Harvey J. Cohen and Arati V. Rao, *Editors*

May 2016
Chronic Conditions in Older Adults with Cardiovascular Disease
Cynthia Boyd, James Pacala, and Michael W. Rich, *Editors*

RECENT ISSUES

May 2015
Geriatric Palliative Care
Madeline Leong and Thomas J. Smith, *Editors*

February 2015
Diabetes and Aging
Elsa S. Strotmeyer, *Editor*

November 2014
Medical Implications of Elder Abuse and Neglect
Lisa M. Gibbs and Laura Mosqueda, *Editors*

ISSUE OF RELATED INTEREST

Medical Clinics of North America March 2015 (Vol. 99, No. 2)
Geriatric Medicine
Susan E. Merel and Jeffrey Wallace, *Editors*
http://www.medical.theclinics.com/

Preface

Novel Approaches to Nutrition in Older Persons

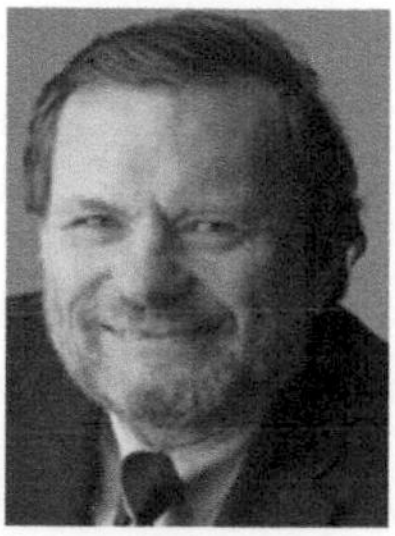

John E. Morley, MB, BCh
Editor

This issue of *Clinics in Geriatric Medicine* recognizes the unique nutrient needs of older persons. Over the last decade, there has been increased recognition of the need for aggressive prevention of weight loss in older persons.[1] This has been highlighted by an improved understanding of the physiologic reasons older persons develop an anorexia of aging.[2] Peripheral hormones, such as cholecystokinin and leptin, and a variety of central neurotransmitters, which modulate the nitric oxide–AMP kinase feeding pathway, are altered with aging. These factors, coupled with the decline in food intake, cause older persons to develop a hypodipsia, which increases their risk of becoming dehydrated when they develop a fever or tachypnea.

It is now well-recognized that the key geriatric syndrome in older persons is "frailty."[3] Malnutrition is one of the causes of frailty. However, the major cause is sarcopenia, the age-related loss of muscle mass.[4] Central to the treatment of sarcopenia is resistance exercise, vitamin D, and protein. Diabetes mellitus has been shown to be a major cause of sarcopenia and frailty.[5] This appears to be predominantly due to insulin resistance, resulting in decreased muscle mitochondrial function and an increase in triglycerides in muscle leading to obese sarcopenia.

An important emerging concept in nutrition is that it is a well-balanced diet rather than individual nutrients that is important. Thus, antioxidant vitamins appear to have a number of negative effects, but when eaten as part of fruits and vegetables, they have shown epidemiologically to markedly improve cognition and extend physiologic life span. The FINGER study has shown that a Mediterranean diet, together with exercise and brain games, results in improved cognitive function in older persons.[6] Multiple other studies have supported the importance of nutrition together with exercise in slowing the cognitive decline that occurs with aging.[7]

Clin Geriatr Med 31 (2015) xiii–xiv
http://dx.doi.org/10.1016/j.cger.2015.05.001

All of these new concepts in nutritional care of older persons are covered in depth in this issue of the *Clinics in Geriatric Medicine*.

John E. Morley, MB, BCh
Divisions of Geriatric Medicine and Endocrinology
Saint Louis University School of Medicine
1402 South Grand Boulevard, M238
St Louis, MO 63104, USA

E-mail address:
morley@slu.edu

REFERENCES

1. Soenen S, Chapman IM. Body weight, anorexia, and undernutrition in older people. J Am Med Dir Assoc 2013;14:642–8.
2. Tamura BK, Bell CL, Masaki KH, et al. Factors associated with weight loss, low BMI, and malnutrition among nursing home patients: a systematic review of the literature. J Am Med Dir Assoc 2013;14:649–55.
3. Morley JE, Vellas B, van Kan GA, et al. Frailty consensus: a call to action. J Am Med Dir Assoc 2013;14:392–7.
4. Fielding RA, Vellas B, Evans WJ, et al. Sarcopenia: an undiagnosed condition in older adults. Current consensus definition: prevalence, etiology, and consequences. international working group on sarcopenia. J Am Med Dir Assoc 2011;12:249–56.
5. Morley JE, Malmstrom TK, Rodriguez-Mañas L, et al. Frailty, sarcopenia and diabetes. J Am Med Dir Assoc 2014;15:853–9.
6. Ngandu T, Lehtisalo J, Solomon A, et al. A 2 year multidomain intervention of diet, exercise, cognitive training, and vascular risk monitoring versus control to prevent cognitive decline in at-risk elderly people (FINGER): a randomized controlled trial. Lancet 2015. http://dx.doi.org/10.1016/S0140-6736(15)60461-5.
7. Shah R. The role of nutrition and diet in Alzheimer disease: a systematic review. J Am Med Dir Assoc 2013;14:398–402.

Excessive Body Weight in Older Adults

Kathryn N. Porter Starr, PhD, RD[a,b,*], Connie W. Bales, PhD, RD[a,b]

KEYWORDS

- Obesity • Overweight • Body mass index • Physical function • Muscle mass
- Weight reduction • Weight maintenance

KEY POINTS

- Obesity is common in older adults, contributing to significant morbidity and reducing functional independence and quality of life.
- Older adults with a body mass index (BMI) less than 23 kg/m^2 are advised to emphasize a diet of high energy and nutrient density and participate in exercise (resistance) training to achieve a gradual increase in body mass, especially muscle mass.
- Older adults who are overweight (BMI 25–29.9 kg/m^2) are advised to remain weight stable, emphasize a diet of high nutrient density, and actively participate in exercise training that enhances aerobic endurance and improves muscle mass.
- For adults aged 60 to 79 years who are obese (BMI >30 kg/m^2) and experiencing metabolic and/or functional deficits, a weight loss therapy that minimizes muscle and bone losses can be beneficial. This therapy should be a combination of calorie reduction and exercise training that includes resistance exercise.
- In the case of obese adults who are older than 79 years or those who have serious chronic illness or disabilities, a weight maintenance approach is best advised, given the scarcity of information about the benefit/risk of weight reduction in these situations.

INTRODUCTION: NATURE OF THE PROBLEM

The pervasiveness of the obesity epidemic in the older adult population is poorly recognized and understudied. Yet, as illustrated in **Fig. 1**, more than one-third of US adults 60 years or older have body weights in the obese (BMI $\geq$30 kg/m^2) range[1]; the prevalence of geriatric obesity has steadily increased in recent decades and is expected to continue to increase.[2] Obesity, inactivity, and aging are each independent risk factors for detrimental metabolic changes leading to conditions such as cardiovascular disease

Disclosures: CW Bales' disclosures include Claude D. Pepper Older Americans Independence Center P30 AG028716 (PI, Cohen); Taylor & Francis, National Pork Board. KN Porter Starr disclosures include NIH 5T32 AG000029 (PI, Cohen).

[a] Department of Medicine, Duke University Medical Center, Box 3003, Durham, NC 27710, USA; [b] Durham VA Medical Center, Geriatric Research, Education and Clinical Center, 508 Fulton Street, Durham, NC 27710, USA

* Corresponding author. Duke University Medical Center, Box 3003, Durham, NC 27710.
E-mail address: kathryn.starr@dm.duke.edu

Clin Geriatr Med 31 (2015) 311–326
http://dx.doi.org/10.1016/j.cger.2015.04.001
0749-0690/15/$ – see front matter Published by Elsevier Inc.

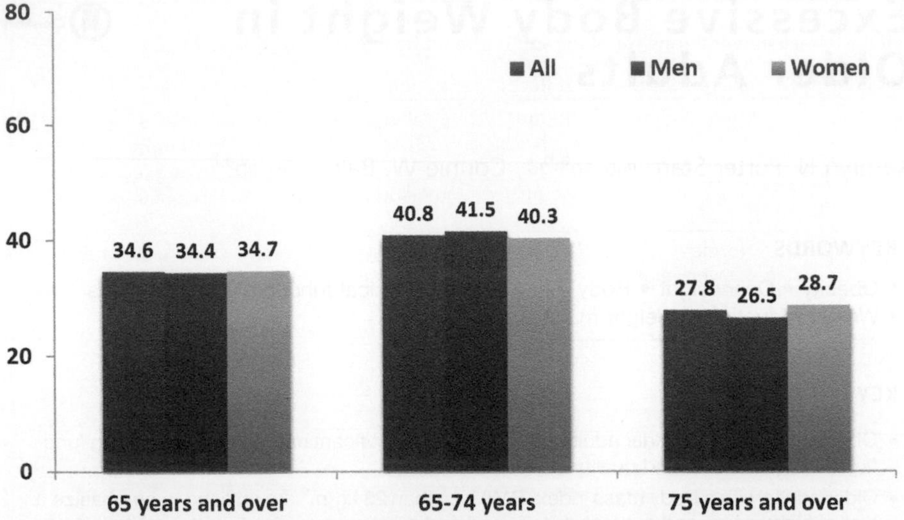

Fig. 1. Prevalence of obesity among adults 65 years and older, by sex: United States 2007–2010. (*From* Fakhouri TH, Ogden CL, Carroll MD, et al. Prevalence of obesity among older adults in the United States, 2007–2010. NCHS data brief, no 106. Hyattsville (MD): National Center for Health Statistics; 2012.)

and impaired glucose intolerance, so the obese older person is especially vulnerable to such derangements.[3,4] However, loss of function is often the most distressful to elders because it threatens independence and dignity during the later years of life.[5–7] These "fat and frail" older adults have insufficient muscle strength relative to body size to remain fully active. The contribution of obesity to impaired function is progressive, as excessive adiposity and loss of muscle strength/mass are cyclically reinforcing.[8]

THERAPEUTIC OPTIONS FOR OPTIMIZING BODY MASS

Table 1 lists categories of BMI level and corresponding lifestyle (diet and exercise) recommendations to optimize health and longevity in older adults based on the best evidence currently available.

Underweight

For older adults, a BMI in the range of 23.0 to 29.9 kg/m^2 is associated with optimal longevity.[9,10] A meta-analysis by Winter and colleagues[9] indicated that, within the normal weight category of 18 to 24.9 kg/m^2, mortality was better at a BMI $\geq$23.0 kg/m^2. Therefore, the authors recommend that older adults with a BMI less than 23.0 kg/m^2 be encouraged to use a combination of nutrient- and calorie-dense foods and exercise to gradually increase their BMI, ideally using resistance training to increase muscle mass.

Overweight

In the case of older adults, a BMI in the range typically categorized as overweight (25.0–29.9 kg/m^2) is not associated with adverse mortality outcomes.[11] Flegal and colleagues[10] analyzed 97 studies (of 2.88 million individuals) and found that being overweight was associated with the lowest mortality across all age groups, as well as in older adults specifically. In their analysis, being obese (BMI $\geq$30 kg/m^2) was associated with higher mortality across all ages, although not in older adults. These findings indicate that

Table 1
Lifestyle recommendations for older adults should be individualized by BMI and age

BMI (kg/m²)	Weight Status	Diet Recommendation	Exercise Recommendation
<23.0	Underweight	High-nutrient-dense diet with sufficient kilocalories to gradually increase weight and muscle mass	Emphasize resistance training to build muscle; also aerobic exercise, balance, and flexibility training
23.0 to 29.9	Normal/ Overweight	High-nutrient-dense diet with sufficient kilocalories to maintain weight	Combination of aerobic exercise, resistance, balance, and flexibility training
≥30, Age ≤80	Obese	Modest calorie reduction (500 to <1000) to achieve gradual weight loss; emphasize high nutrient density	Combination of aerobic exercise, resistance, balance, and flexibility training
≥30, Age >80	Obese	High-nutrient-dense diet with sufficient kilocalories to maintain weight	Resistance, balance, and flexibility training; aerobic exercise as tolerated

the protective effects of overweight on survival occur independently of age and that in the case of obesity detrimental effects on survival are somewhat blunted in later life.

Obese, Younger Than 80 Years

Until recently, weight reduction therapies for obesity in older adults have been deemed controversial.[12–14] With traditional weight loss regimens, the loss of lean muscle mass can constitute 25% or more of the total amount of weight lost.[15] Bone mineral density is also slightly reduced when weight loss occurs.[12] Thus, there is tension between the need to minimize the negative side effects of weight loss and the many advantages of reducing excess body weight. However, for older adults who are obese and experiencing metabolic or functional challenges, recent evidence argues that beneficial and safe body weight reduction can be achieved, especially when exercise is included as part of the treatment.[16] Based on studies in obese older adults who are physically able to participate, both aerobic and resistance exercise training can help to protect lean mass and preserve function during weight loss.[17–19] Although weight loss interventions for older adults remain controversial, per the accumulating evidence from randomized controlled trials illustrated in the next section, weight reduction in this population can benefit muscle quality, physical function, inflammatory status, and metabolic profiles.[2,12,16]

Obese, Older Than 80 Years or with Complicating Circumstances

There are essentially no studies of obesity reduction in adults 80 years of age or older. In these individuals, the authors therefore advocate for weight maintenance, with an emphasis on a healthy diet and exercise as tolerated; this would also be the case for any older adult with a terminal illness, those with severe chronic medical conditions, and persons with moderate to severe dementia.

CLINICAL OUTCOMES

Weight loss therapy that minimizes loss of muscle and bone mass is recommended for older persons who are obese and who have functional impairments or medical complications that can benefit from weight reduction.[20] **Table 2**

Table 2
Nonpharmacologic weight loss interventions

Studies	Study Population	Intervention	Outcomes	Important Findings
Beavers et al,[30] 2015	N = 24 Mean age: 68.4 ± 5.5 y Gender: 88% women BMI: 35.1 ± 4.3 kg/m^2 Health: Abdominal obesity (WC ≥102 men 88 cm for men and women)	Design: RCT Arms: WL+soy (n = 12) WL+non-soy (n = 12) Control (n = 93) Duration: 3 mo	Body composition by DXA; cardiometabolic biomarkers (systolic and diastolic BP, glucose, serum insulin, total cholesterol, triglycerides, LDL, HDL, and HsCRP); SPPB; 400-m walk; knee extensor strength using dynamometer; grip strength	Weight change: WL+soy: −7.2 ± 7.8 kg; WL+non-soy: −8.4 ± 3.7 kg Body composition: No difference between arms on all body composition measures. All body composition measures were significantly decreased in both groups except thigh intermuscular fat volume. Total body fat was reduced by 5.3 ± 2.4 kg and lean mass by 2.5 ± 1.9 kg in both arms combined Function: No difference between interventions. Combined, there was no change in 400-m walk time, SPPB, and grip strength; knee extensor strength was significantly reduced (−5.09 ± 9.4 N/m). When knee extensor strength was corrected for thigh muscle volume there, was no longer a significant change (−0.00 ± 0.02 N/m) Cardiometabolic biomarkers: Diastolic BP was significantly reduced in the WL+non-soy group (66.7 ± 2.7 mm Hg) compared with WL+soy group (75.3 ± 2.7 mm Hg). No other cardiometabolic biomarkers differed between interventions. Combined, both interventions had significant reductions in systolic BP (−9.4 ± 45.6 mm Hg), total cholesterol (−24.6 ± 20.6 mg/dL), LDL (−14.0 ± 20.0 mg/dL), and insulin (−4.4 ± 6.0 μIU/mL) measures
Verreijen et al,[24] 2015	N = 60 Mean age: 63.0 ± 5.6 y Gender: 53% women BMI: 33.0 ± 4.4 kg/m^2 Health: BMI ≥30 kg/m^2 or BMI ≥28 kg/m^2 and abdominal obesity (WC ≥102 men 88 cm for men and women)	Design: RCT Arms: EX+WL+protein (n = 30) EX+WL (n = 30) Duration: 13 wk	Body composition by DXA; handgrip strength; 4-m gait speed; 400-m walk speed; chair strength	Weight change: WL+protein+EX: −3.4 ± 3.6 kg; WL+EX: −2.8 ± 2.8 kg, no difference between arms Body composition: Fat mass was decreased in both arms (WL+protein+EX: −3.2 ± 3.1 kg; WL+EX: −2.5 ± 2.4 kg). Appendicular and leg muscle mass differed between arms (WL+protein+EX: 0.4 ± 1.2 kg; 0.3 ± 1.2 kg vs WL+EX: −0.5 ± 2.1 kg; −0.6 ± 1.2 kg) Function: No difference between interventions. All functional measures significantly improved in both arms

Beavers et al,[31] 2014; Beavers et al,[32] 2013; Rejeski et al,[33] 2011	N = 288 Mean age: 67 ± 5 y Gender: 67% women BMI: 32.8 ± 3.8 kg/m² Health: CVD or cardiometabolic dysfunction and self-reported functional limitations	Design: RCT Arms: WL+EX (n = 98) EX (n = 97) Control (n = 93) Duration: 18 mo	Body composition by DXA; cardiometabolic biomarkers (systolic and diastolic BP, glucose, serum insulin, total cholesterol, triglycerides, LDL, HDL, HOMA-IR); inflammatory markers (adiponectin, leptin, high-sensitivity IL-6, IL6sR, and sTNFR1); 400-m walk	Weight change: WL+EX: −7.3 ± 7.1 kg; EX: −1.3 ± 5.1 kg; Control: −1.0 ± 6.2 kg Body composition: Fat mass was significantly reduced in the WL+EX arm compared with EX and Control arms. Lean mass decreased greater in WL+EX arm (−2.5 ± 2.8 kg) compared with EX (−0.7 ± 2.2 kg) and Control (−0.8 ± 2.4 kg) arms Function: Walking speed increased more in WL+EX (323.3 [3.7] s) compared with EX (336.3 [3.9] s) and Control (341.3 [3.9] s) arms Cardiometabolic biomarkers: Decreased body mass was significantly associated with improvements in diastolic BP, triglycerides, glucose, insulin, HOMA-IR, and HDL Inflammatory biomarkers: Leptin and hsIL-6 levels were significantly lower in WL+EX (21.3 [19.7, 22.9] ng/mL; 2.1 [1.9, 2.3] pg/mL) compared with EX (29.3 [26.9, 31.8] ng/mL; 2.5 [2.3, 2.7] pg/mL) and Control (30.3 [27.9, 32.8] ng/mL; 2.4 [2.2, 2.6] pg/mL) arms
Beavers et al,[34] 2014	N = 284 Mean age: 66 ± 6 y Gender: 67% women BMI: 33.4 ± 3.7 kg/m² Health: OA in one or both knees	Design: RCT Arms: WL+EX (n = 101) WL (n = 88) EX (n = 95) Duration: 18 mo	Regional BMD and T-scores at hip and spine; body composition by DXA	Weight change: WL+EX: −10.4 ± 8.0 kg; WL: −9.1 ± 8.6 kg; EX: −1.3 ± 4.5 kg BMD: Significant reduction in BMD at hip and femoral neck in both WL+EX (−19.5 [−25.8, −13.2]; −12.5 [−18.1, −6.8]) and WL (−23.7 [−30.3, −17.2]; −13.2 [−19.1, −7.3]) arms compared with EX (−2.0 [−8.5, 4.4]; −0.8 [−6.6, 5.0])
Solomon et al,[35] 2013	N = 15 Mean age: 65 ± 1 y Gender: 55% women BMI: 35.0 ± 1.0 kg/m² Health: Sedentary	Design: RCT Arms: WL low GI+EX (n = 4) WL high GI+EX (n = 11) Duration: 3 mo	Muscle lipid composition by ^{3}H-MRS of soleus muscle	Weight change: −8.6 ± 1.1% for both groups Muscle lipid composition: Unchanged

(*continued on next page*)

Table 2
(continued)

Studies	Study Population	Intervention	Outcomes	Important Findings
Armamento-Villareal et al,[36] 2012; Villareal et al,[16] 2011; Shah et al,[37] 2011	N = 93 Age: Control: 69 ± 4 y; WL, EX, and WL+EX:70 ± 4 y Gender: Control: 67% women; WL: 65% women; EX: 62% women; WL+EX: 57% women BMI: Control: 37.3 ± 4.7; WL: 37.2 ± 4.5; EX: 36.9 ± 5.4; WL+EX: 37.2 ± 5.4 kg/m^2 Health: Mild to moderate frailty Sedentary lifestyle	Design: RCT Arms: Control (n = 27) WL (n = 26) EX (n = 26) WL+EX (n = 28) Duration: 12 mo	BMD; serum sclerostin; hip geometry; C-terminal telopeptide of type collagen 1; osteocalcin; N-terminal propeptide of type 1 procollagen, serum estradiol, IGF-1; vitamin D; serum PTH; PPT; Vo_2 max; FSQ score; 1-RM; dynamic balance (obstacle course); static balance (single limb leg stance time); gait speed; SF-36; body composition by DXA; anthropometrics	Weight change: Control: −0.1 ± 3.5 kg, <1%; WL: −9.7 ± 5.4 kg, 10%; EX: −0.5 ± 3.6 kg, 1%; WL+EX: −8.6 ± 3.8 kg, 9% Function: WL+EX and EX arms significantly improved in all functional measures compared with control. WL significantly improved compared with control in all functional measures except strength and gait speed. PPT and Vo_2 improved more in WL+EX than WL or EX. Similar improvements were seen between WL+EX and EX arms in FSQ, 1-RM and gait speed, and between WL+EX and WL in single limb leg stance time Body composition: Significant and similar decrease in BW and FM in WL and WL+EX arm. FFM increased in EX and decreased less in the WL+EX group compared with WL BMD: Increased in EX (1.5 ± 1.6%) and decreased in WL (−2.6 ± 2.1%) and WL+EX (−1.1 ± 2.7%) Bone metabolism: Sclerostin level increased in diet arm (10.5 ± 1.9%) and unchanged in all other arms. Serum CTX and osteocalcin levels increased in the WL arm (24 ± 32%), decreased in the EX arm (−13 ± 31%), and remained unchanged in the WL+EX arm. Serum 25(OH)D level increased in all arms. Serum leptin and estradiol levels remained unchanged in EX and control arms, but decreased in the WL (−25 ± 31%; −15 ± 18%) and WL+EX (−38 ± 26%; −13 ± 30%), arms Hip geometry: Significant decreases in cross-sectional area and cortical thickness and increases in bucking ratio at narrow neck, intertrochanter and femoral shaft in all arms except WL-EX arm

Anton et al,[17] 2011	N = 34 Age: 63.7 ± 4.5 y Gender: Women only BMI: Control: 35.8 ± 6.8 kg/m^2, WL+EX: 37.8 ± 5.5 kg/m^2 Health: Mild to moderate functional impairment	Design: RCT Arms: Control (n = 17) WL+EX (n = 17) Duration: 6 mo	Walking speed; SPPB; knee extension isokinetic; anthropometrics	Weight change: Control: −0.23 ± 4.08 kg; WL+EX:−5.95 ± 4.08 kg Function: Walking speed increased more in WL+EX compared with control (0.16 ± 0.03 m/s vs 0.02 ± 0.03 m/s); WL+EX and control increased SPPB scores, with greater increase in WL+EX (1.82 ± 1.24 vs 0.80 ± 1.20) Other: WL+EX decreased BW greater than control (5.95 ± 0.992 vs 0.23 ± 0.99 kg)
Dube et al,[38] 2011	N = 16 Mean age: 67.2 ± 4.0 y Gender: 56.2% women BMI: 30.6 ± 0.8 kg/m^2 Health: Impaired glucose tolerance or elevated fasting blood glucose	Design: RCT Arms: Aerobic EX (n = 8) WL (n = 8) Duration: 4 mo	Muscle lipid composition by histochemistry of muscle biopsy Body composition by DXA	Weight change: WL: −8.5 ± 1.5%; EX: −1.8 ± 0.9% Muscle lipid composition: Decreased in WL (−16.0 ± 3.2%); increased in EX (40.8 ± 18.2%) Body composition: Fat mass decreased greater in WL than in EX. FFM decreased in WL, increased slightly in EX
Haus et al,[39] 2011	N = 36 Mean age: 66 ± 1 y Gender: 83.3% women BMI: 32.9 ± 3.2 kg/m^2 Health: Sedentary	Design: RCT Arms: WL low GI+EX (n = 7) WL high GI+EX (n = 8) Duration: 7 d	Muscle lipid composition by ^{3}H-MRS of soleus muscle	Weight change: WL low GI+EX: −1.7 ± 0.6 kg; WL high GI+EX: −1.9 ± 0.6 Muscle lipid composition: Increased, 2.3+1.3 mmol/kg in WL low GI+EX and 1.4 ± 0.9 in WL high GI+EX. No group difference found
Kelly et al,[40] 2011	N = 28 Mean age: 66 ± 1 y Gender: 83.3% women BMI: 34.2 ± 0.7 kg/m^2 Health: Insulin-resistant; sedentary	Design: RCT Arms: WL low GI+EX (n = 13) WL high GI+EX (n = 15) Duration: 3 mo	Plasma and MNC TNF-α; IL-6; MCP-1; glucose; insulin; HbA1c; body composition via DXA	Weight change: WL low GI+EX −6.5 kg; WL high GI+EX:−9.6; no significant difference between arms Cardiometabolic biomarkers: Significant reduction in fasting plasma glucose and insulin levels in both arms. Oral glucose tolerance was only reduced in the WL low GI+EX arm Inflammatory biomarkers: MNC and plasma TNF-α levels were reduced in the WL low GI+EX arm and increased in the WL high GI+EX arm. Plasma IL-6 level was reduced in both arms with a significantly greater reduction in the WL low GI+EX arm Body composition: Fat mass and fat-free mass were both significantly reduced in both arms, no difference between arms

(*continued on next page*)

Table 2
(continued)

Studies	Study Population	Intervention	Outcomes	Important Findings
Santanasto et al,[41] 2011	N = 36 Mean age: 70.3 ± 5.9 y Gender: 83.3% women BMI: 32.9 ± 3.2 kg/m^2 Health: Sedentary	Design: RCT Arms: WL+EX (n = 21) EX+Edu (n = 15) Duration: 6 mo	Muscle lipid composition by CT of thigh; CT of abdomen; body composition by DXA; anthropometrics; SPPB; knee extensor strength, CHAMPS questionnaire	Weight change: −4.9 ± 4.8 kg in WL+EX;−1.0 ± 3.5 kg in EX+Edu Muscle lipid composition: *Decreased in thigh of both groups,* −18.1 ± 17.5 cm in WL+EX and −5.4 ± 9.9 cm in EX+Edu, but group effect *P*<.07 Body composition: WL+EX decreased body fat, FFM, subcutaneous total visceral fat, SAT, VAT, and thigh fat, waist circumference and knee extensor strength and increased SPPB score
Chomentowski et al,[42] 2009	N = 29 Age: 67.2 ± 4.2 Gender: 55.2% women BMI: 31.8 ± 3.3 kg/m^2 Health: Impaired fasting glucose tolerance, impaired fasting glucose, or drug-naive type 2 diabetes; sedentary	Design: RCT Arms: WL+EX (n = 18) WL (n = 11) Duration: 4 mo	Body composition by DXA; thigh muscle cross-sectional area by CT scan; skeletal muscle fiber size	Weight change: WL+EX: −9.2% ± 1.0%; WL: −9.1% ± 1.0% Body composition: BW and total fat mass significantly decreased in both arms. WL (−4.3% ± 1.2%) lost significantly more lean mass compared with WL+EX (−1.1% ± 1.0%) CSA: Thigh muscle decreased in both arms Muscle fiber: Type 1 and II muscle fiber area significantly decreased in WL (−19.2% ± 7.9%; −16.6% ± 4.0%), but not in WL+EX (3.4% ± 7.5%; −0.2% ± 6.5%)
Davidson et al,[43] 2009	N = 117 Age: Women: 67.4 ± 5.1 y; Men: 67.7 ± 5.1 y Gender: 58.0% women BMI: Women: 30.5 ± 2.0 kg/m^2; men: 30.4 ± 2.7 kg/m^2 Health: Abdominal obesity, Sedentary	Design: RCT Arms: Control (n = 28) Resistance EX (n = 36) Aerobic EX (n = 37) Combined EX (n = 35) Duration: 6 mo	Chair stands; 2-min step; 8-ft-up-and-go; seated arm curl; Vo_2 max; anthropometrics; body composition by MRI	Weight change: Control: 0.28 ± 0.37 kg; resistance EX: −0.64 ± 0.37 kg; aerobic EX: −2.77 ± 0.33 kg; combined EX: −2.31 ± 0.33 kg Function: Chair stands; 2-min step; 8-ft-up-and-go; seated arm curl improved in all EX arms, with combined EX having greater improvements than aerobic EX. Vo_2 increased in aerobic EX and combined EX Body composition: BW and total fat decreased in aerobic and combined EX compared with control and resistance EX arms. Abdominal fat level decreased in aerobic EX and combined EX compared with control only; FFM increased in resistance EX ad combined EX compared with control and aerobic EX

Frimel et al,[18] 2008	N = 30 Age: WL: 70.3 ± 4.8 y; WL+EX: 68.7 ± 4.3 y Gender: 60% women BMI: WL: 36.9 ± 4.9 kg/m²; WL+EX:36.7 ± 5.1 kg/m² Health: Mild to moderate frailty; sedentary	Design: RCT Arms: WL (n = 15) WL+EX (n = 15) Duration: 6 mo	1-RM; body composition by DXA; anthropometrics	Weight change: WL: −10.7 ± 4.5 kg, 10.6 ± 4.6%; WL+EX: −9.7 ± 4.0 kg, 100 ± 3.9% Function: WL+EX increased in upper and lower extremity strength (1-RM) Body composition: WL and WL+EX decreased BW and FM; WL+EX lost less FFM (1.8 ± 1.5 vs 5.4 ± 3.7 kg), and upper (0.1 ± 0.2 vs 0.2 ± 0.2 kg) and lower (0.9 ± 0.8 vs 2.0 ± 0.9 kg) extremity FFM compared with WL arm
Lambert et al,[44] 2008	N = 16 Age: 69 ± 1 y Gender: EX: 50% women; WL: 50% women BMI: 38 ± 2 kg/m² Health: Frail; difficulty or need for assistance in 2 IADLS of 1 ADL	Design: RCT Arms: EX WL Duration: 12 wk	Skeletal muscle mRNAs for toll-like receptor-4; mechano-growth factor, TNF-α; IL-6; HsCRP: body composition via DXA	Weight change: WL: 7.1%; EX: 0% Inflammation/ROS biomarkers: EX decreased TLR-4 mRNA; IL-6 mRNA; TNF-α mRNA; EX increased MGF mRNA
Solomon et al,[45] 2008	N = 23 Mean age: 66 ± 1 y Gender: Both BMI: 33.2 ± 1.4 kg/m² Health: Impaired glucose tolerance	Design: RCT Arms: EX (n = 12) WL+EX (n = 11) Duration: 12 wk	Muscle lipid composition by histochemistry of muscle biopsy; body composition by hydrostatic weighing; anthropometrics	Weight change: EX: −3.3 kg; WL+EX: −7.9 kg Muscle lipid composition: Decreased −25.9 ± 12.4% in EX and −34.3 ± 17.6% in WL+EX, no group difference found Body composition: No change in FFM. WL+EX had greater decreases in body and fat mass

(*continued on next page*)

Table 2
(continued)

Studies	Study Population	Intervention	Outcomes	Important Findings
Villareal et al,[46] 2008	N = 27 Mean age: 70 ± 5 y Gender: Both BMI: 39 ± 5 kg/m^2 Health: Sedentary; mild to moderate frailty defined by physical performance score, peak Vo_2, and IADLS and ADL	Design: RCT Arms: WL+EX (n = 17) Control (n = 10) Duration: 1 y	BW, BMD, BMC, bone metabolism markers, and strength assessed by 1-RM	Weight change: WL+EX: −10.1 ± 2.0%; Control: +1.2 ± 1.3% BMD: Decreased greater in WL+EX arm compared with control at total hip (−2.4 ± 2.5% vs 0.1 ± 2.1%), trochanter (−3.3 ± 3.1% vs 0.2 ± 3.3%), and intertrochanter (−2.7 ± 3.0% 0.3 ± 2.7%) BMC: Decreased greater in WL+EX compared with control arm at total hip (−2.4 ± 4.7% vs 0.9 ± 2.0%), trochanter (−4.1 ± 7.0% vs 1.4 ± 6.1%), and intertrochanter (−2.4 ± 5.7% vs 0.6 ± 2.0%) Bone markers: Greater increase in WL+EX arm compared with control in C-terminal telopeptide (101 ± 79% vs 12 ± 35%) and osteocalcin (66 ± 61% vs −5 ± 15%) Hormones: Decreased greater in WL+EX compared with control arm in serum leptin (−30 ± 25% vs 2 ± 12%) and estradiol (−14 ± 21% vs 0/1 ± 14%) Strength: Significant improvements in upper and lower body compared with control
Miller et al,[47] 2006	N = 87 Age: Control: 69.3 ± 0.9 y; WL+EX: 69.7 ± 0.9 y Gender: WS: 60.5% women; WL+EX: 63.6% BMI: Control: 34.3 ± 3.9 kg/m^2; WL: 34.9 ± 4.9 kg/m^2 Health: Symptomatic knee OA; difficulty with 1 or more: lifting and carrying groceries, walking one-quarter mile, getting in and out of a chair, or going up and down stairs	Design: RCT Arms: Control (n = 43) WL+EX (n = 44) Duration: 6 mo	WOMAC; 6-min walk distance test; stair climb test; body composition by DXA; anthropometrics	Weight change: Control: −0.1 ± 0.7 kg; WL+EX: −8.3 ± 0.7 kg Function: Compared with control WL+EX had improvements in WOMAC score in WL+EX; walking distance; faster stair climb in WL+EX Body composition: BW, WC, FM, and FFM decreased in WL+EX compared with control

Villareal et al,[48] 2006	N = 27 Age: Control: 71.1 ± 5.1 y; WL+EX: 69.4 ± 4.6 y Gender: Both BMI: Control: 39.0 ± 5.0 kg/m^2; WL+EX: 38.5 ± 5.3 kg/m^2 Health: Mild to moderate frailty	Design: RCT Arms: Control (n = 10) WL+EX (n = 17) Duration: 6 mo	PPT; Vo_2 max; FSQ score; 1-RM; knee extensor and flexor strength; dynamic balance (obstacle course); static balance (single limb leg stance time); gait speed; SF-36; body composition by DXA; anthropometrics	Weight change: Control: 0.7 ± 2.7 kg; WL+EX: −8.2 ± 5.7 kg Function: WL+EX inc; Vo_2; FSQ score; knee extension and flexor strength; gait speed; physical function (SF-36); role limitations (SF-36); bodily pain (SF-36); vitality (SF-36), and change in health (SF-36). WL+EX improved one leg limb stand and obstacle course time Body composition: BW and FM decreased in WL+EX. No difference between FFM loss in control and WL+EX
Messier et al,[49] 2004	N = 252 Age: Healthy lifestyle: 69 ± 0.1 y; WL: 68 ± 0.7 y; EX: 69 ± 0.8 y; WL+EX: 69 ± 0.8 y Gender: Control: 68% women; WL: 72% women; EX: 74% women; WL+EX: 74% women BMI: Control: 34.2 ± 0.6 kg/m^2; WL: 34.5 ± 0.6 kg/m^2; EX: 34.2 ± 0.6 kg/m^2; WL+EX: 34.0 ± 0.7 kg/m^2 Health: Knee pain, radiographic evidence of knee OA, sedentary, self-reported physical disability	Design: RCT Arms: Control (n = 78) WL (n = 82) EX (n = 80) WL+EX (n = 76) Duration: 18 mo	WOMAC; 6-min walk; timed stair-climb; Body composition by DXA; anthropometrics	Weight change: Control: 1.2% WL: 4.5%; EX: 3.7%; WL+EX: 5.7% Function: WL+EX decreased WOMAC score compared with control; WL+EX and WL decreased WOMAC score compared with baseline scores. 6-min walk distance increased in WL+EX and EX compared with control and stair-climb time decreased in WL+EX Body composition: WL+EX and WL decreased in BW compared with control

(*continued on next page*)

Table 2
(continued)

Studies	Study Population	Intervention	Outcomes	Important Findings
Nicklas et al,[50] 2004	N = 252 Age: Control: 69 ± 0.1 y; WL: 68 ± 0.7 y; EX: 69 ± 0.8 y; WL+EX: 69 ± 0.8 y Gender: Control: 68% women; WL: 72% women; EX: 74% women; WL+EX: 74% women BMI: Control: 34.2 ± 0.6 kg/m^2; diet only: 34.5 ± 0.6 kg/m^2; EX only: 34.2 ± 0.6 kg/m^2; WL+EX: 34.0 ± 0.7 kg/m^2 Health: Knee pain, radiographic evidence of knee OA, sedentary, self-reported physical disability	Design: RCT Arms: Control WL EX WL+EX Duration: 18 mo	IL-6; TNF-α; IL-6sR; sTNFR1; sTNFR2; CRP	Weight change: Control: 2.3% WL: 12.8%; EX: 4.1%; WL+EX: 8.2% Inflammation/ROS biomarkers: WL decreased C-reactive protein, IL-6, and sTNFR1. Decreases in sTNFR1 correlated with decreases in BW

Abbreviations: 1-RM, 1 repetition maximum; ADL, activities of daily living; Anthropometrics, body weight, height, BMI, waist circumference; BMC, bone mineral content; BMD, bone mineral density; BP, blood pressure; BW, body weight; CHAMPS, Community Health Activities Model Program for Seniors physical activity questionnaire; CRP, C-reactive protein; CT, computed tomography; CTX, cross-linked C-telopeptide; CVD, cardiovascular disease; DXA, duel energy X-ray absorptiometry; EX, exercise intervention; EX+Edu, exercise and health education intervention; FFM, fat-free mass; FM, fat mass; FSQ, functional status questionnaire; GI, glycemic index; HDL, high-density lipoprotein; ^{3}H-MRS, proton magnetic resonance spectroscopy; HOMA-IR, homeostasis model assessment of insulin resistance; HsCRP, high-sensitivity C-reactive protein; IADL, instrumental activities of daily living; IGF-1, insulin-like growth factor 1; IL-6, interleukin-6; IL-6sR, soluble IL-6 receptor; LDL, low-density lipoprotein; MGF, mechano-growth factor; MNC, mononuclear cells; OA, osteoarthritis; PPT, physical performance test; PTH, parathyroid hormone; RCT, randomized control trial; ROS, reactive oxygen species; SAT, subcutaneous adipose tissue; SF-36, short form health survey; soy, soy protein; SPPB, short physical performance battery; sTNFR1, soluble TNF-α receptor 1; sTNFR2, soluble TNF-α receptor 2; TLR-4, toll-like receptor-4; VAT, visceral adipose tissue; Vo_2 max, cardiorespiratory fitness; WC, waist circumference; WL, weight loss intervention; WL+EX, weight loss and exercise intervention; WOMAC, Western Ontario and McMaster Universities Osteoarthritis Index.

Data from Refs.[16–18,24,30–50]

presents the findings to date of clinical intervention trials for obesity reduction in older adults.

COMPLICATIONS AND CONCERNS

The best solution for halting cyclic and progressive functional and metabolic deterioration in those obese older adults with complicated health concerns awaits further study before evidence-based recommendations can be made. For individuals who are able, the use of physical activity, specifically resistance exercise, seems to be the best approach to protect muscle and bone while undergoing intentional weight loss. Therefore, the authors strongly advocate for the combined approach of a weight-reduction diet plus a program of exercise. However, in the case of the obese, frail, older adult who is unable to achieve a level of physical activity sufficient to provide this protection, the best approach in terms of long-term health impact is unknown.[21] Future studies of generous protein intakes as a means of preserving lean muscle mass during weight reduction may yield guidance on this issue.[20,22–24]

The risk of developing serious chronic health conditions increases with age. Unfortunately, these conditions sometimes lead to pronounced conditions of wasting, also known as cachexia.[25] In these cases, the reverse epidemiology of obesity or obesity paradox is often observed, meaning that those with a high BMI survive longer than those with a lower body weight. This phenomenon has been confirmed in the case of cancer cachexia,[26] end-stage renal disease,[27] and chronic heart failure,[28] as well as several other conditions common in old age. The increased survival attributed to obesity in these situations is thought to be due to the availability of larger body stores of both energy (fat) and lean mass, as well as a better nutritional state overall.[29] Taking into consideration the points made in this section, an individualized approach to obesity, with careful consideration of health and quality-of-life priorities, should be taken in the following situations:

- Disability that precludes physical exercise
- Osteoporosis
- Muscle wasting
- Moderate to advanced dementia
- An ultimately terminal condition
- Disease states that might progress to a state of wasting/cachexia (eg, advanced renal disease, heart failure, chronic obstructive pulmonary disease, certain cancers)

SUMMARY

Biological heterogeneity is a hallmark of aging, and approaches to managing obesity in late life must take into account this heterogeneity. Interventions for restoring optimal body mass need to consider medical history and future health trajectories so that recommendations can be tailored to the needs of the individual. The combination of exercise (particularly resistance training) with a gradual weight-reduction diet is the best means to protect lean muscle mass and bone mineral density during weight loss. This approach is recommended for adults younger than 80 years who are experiencing metabolic and/or functional problems as a result of a BMI of 30 kg/m^2 or more and who are physically able to exercise. For obese adults who are 80 years or older or who have potential contraindications for weight reduction, a regimen of healthy diet plus individualized exercise geared toward weight maintenance and enhanced muscle mass is recommended. Further study is needed to identify the diet and exercise strategies most suitable for overweight older adults, namely, the optimal approaches for preventing the development of obesity and slowing the progression of obesity-related chronic health conditions in this age group. Determination of the optimal body mass and composition for older adults based on the age and health status of the individual continues to be an active area of study in the geriatrics field.

REFERENCES

1. Mathus-Vliegen EM. Obesity and the elderly. J Clin Gastroenterol 2012;46(7): 533–44.
2. Porter Starr KN, McDonald SR, Bales CW. Obesity and physical frailty in older adults: a scoping review of lifestyle intervention trials. J Am Med Dir Assoc 2014;15(4):240–50.
3. Dey DK, Lissner L. Obesity in 70-year-old subjects as a risk factor for 15-year coronary heart disease incidence. Obes Res 2003;11(7):817–27.
4. Fagot-Campagna A, Bourdel-Marchasson I, Simon D. Burden of diabetes in an aging population: prevalence, incidence, mortality, characteristics and quality of care. Diabetes Metab 2005;31(Spec No 2). 5S35–52.
5. Vincent HK, Vincent KR, Lamb KM. Obesity and mobility disability in the older adult. Obes Rev 2010;11(8):568–79.
6. Jensen GL, Hsiao PY. Obesity in older adults: relationship to functional limitation. Curr Opin Clin Nutr Metab Care 2010;13(1):46–51.
7. Naugle KM, Higgins TJ, Manini TM. Obesity and use of compensatory strategies to perform common daily activities in pre-clinically disabled older adults. Arch Gerontol Geriatr 2012;54(2):e134–8.
8. Rolland Y, Lauwers-Cances V, Cristini C, et al. Difficulties with physical function associated with obesity, sarcopenia, and sarcopenic-obesity in community-dwelling elderly women: the EPIDOS (EPIDemiologie de l'OSteoporose) study. Am J Clin Nutr 2009;89(6):1895–900.
9. Winter JE, MacInnis RJ, Wattanapenpaiboon N, et al. BMI and all-cause mortality in older adults: a meta-analysis. Am J Clin Nutr 2014;99(4):875–90.
10. Flegal KM, Kit BK, Graubard BI. Overweight, obesity, and all-cause mortality–reply. JAMA 2013;309(16):1681–2.
11. Johnson MA, Bales CW. Is there a best body mass index for older adults? Moving closer to evidence-based recommendations regarding "overweight," health, and mortality. J Nutr Gerontol Geriatr 2014;33(1):1–9.
12. Waters DL, Ward AL, Villareal DT. Weight loss in obese adults 65years and older: a review of the controversy. Exp Gerontol 2013;48(10):1054–61.
13. Decaria JE, Sharp C, Petrella RJ. Scoping review report: obesity in older adults. Int J Obes (Lond) 2012;36(9):1141–50.
14. Darmon P. Intentional weight loss in older adults: useful or wasting disease generating strategy? Curr Opin Clin Nutr Metab Care 2013;16(3):284–9.
15. Weinheimer EM, Sands LP, Campbell WW. A systematic review of the separate and combined effects of energy restriction and exercise on fat-free mass in middle-aged and older adults: implications for sarcopenic obesity. Nutr Rev 2010;68(7):375–88.
16. Villareal DT, Chode S, Parimi N, et al. Weight loss, exercise, or both and physical function in obese older adults. N Engl J Med 2011;364(13):1218–29.
17. Anton SD, Manini TM, Milsom VA, et al. Effects of a weight loss plus exercise program on physical function in overweight, older women: a randomized controlled trial. Clin Interv Aging 2011;6:141–9.

18. Frimel TN, Sinacore DR, Villareal DT. Exercise attenuates the weight-loss-induced reduction in muscle mass in frail obese older adults. Med Sci Sports Exerc 2008; 40(7):1213–9.
19. Villareal DT, Smith GI, Sinacore DR, et al. Regular multicomponent exercise increases physical fitness and muscle protein anabolism in frail, obese, older adults. Obesity (Silver Spring) 2011;19(2):312–8.
20. Mathus-Vliegen EM, Basdevant A, Finer N, et al. Prevalence, pathophysiology, health consequences and treatment options of obesity in the elderly: a guideline. Obes Facts 2012;5(3):460–83.
21. Miller SL, Wolfe RR. The danger of weight loss in the elderly. J Nutr Health Aging 2008;12(7):487–91.
22. McDonald SR, Porter Starr KN, Mauceri L, et al. Meal-based enhancement of protein quality and quantity during weight loss in obese older adults with mobility limitations: rationale and design for the MEASUR-UP trial. Contemp Clin Trials 2015; 40:112–23.
23. Paddon-Jones D, Leidy H. Dietary protein and muscle in older persons. Curr Opin Clin Nutr Metab Care 2014;17(1):5–11.
24. Verreijen AM, Verlaan S, Engberink MF, et al. A high whey protein-, leucine-, and vitamin D-enriched supplement preserves muscle mass during intentional weight loss in obese older adults: a double-blind randomized controlled trial. Am J Clin Nutr 2015;101(2):279–86.
25. Evans WJ, Morley JE, Argiles J, et al. Cachexia: a new definition. Clin Nutr 2008; 27(6):793–9.
26. Gonzalez MC, Pastore CA, Orlandi SP, et al. Obesity paradox in cancer: new insights provided by body composition. Am J Clin Nutr 2014;99(5):999–1005.
27. Park J, Ahmadi SF, Streja E, et al. Obesity paradox in end-stage kidney disease patients. Prog Cardiovasc Dis 2014;56(4):415–25.
28. Clark AL, Fonarow GC, Horwich TB. Obesity and the obesity paradox in heart failure. Prog Cardiovasc Dis 2014;56(4):409–14.
29. Soeters PB, Sobotka L. The pathophysiology underlying the obesity paradox. Nutrition 2012;28(6):613–5.
30. Beavers KM, Gordon MM, Easter L, et al. Effect of protein source during weight loss on body composition, cardiometabolic risk and physical performance in abdominally obese, older adults: a pilot feeding study. J Nutr Health Aging 2015;19(1):87–95.
31. Beavers KM, Beavers DP, Nesbit BA, et al. Effect of an 18-month physical activity and weight loss intervention on body composition in overweight and obese older adults. Obesity (Silver Spring) 2014;22(2):325–31.
32. Beavers KM, Ambrosius WT, Nicklas BJ, et al. Independent and combined effects of physical activity and weight loss on inflammatory biomarkers in overweight and obese older adults. J Am Geriatr Soc 2013;61(7):1089–94.
33. Rejeski WJ, Brubaker PH, Goff DC Jr, et al. Translating weight loss and physical activity programs into the community to preserve mobility in older, obese adults in poor cardiovascular health. Arch Intern Med 2011;171(10):880–6.
34. Beavers DP, Beavers KM, Loeser RF, et al. The independent and combined effects of intensive weight loss and exercise training on bone mineral density in overweight and obese older adults with osteoarthritis. Osteoarthritis Cartilage 2014;22(6):726–33.
35. Solomon TP, Haus JM, Cook MA, et al. A low-glycemic diet lifestyle intervention improves fat utilization during exercise in older obese humans. Obesity (Silver Spring) 2013;21(11):2272–8.

36. Armamento-Villareal R, Sadler C, Napoli N, et al. Weight loss in obese older adults increases serum sclerostin and impairs hip geometry but both are prevented by exercise training. J Bone Miner Res 2012;27(5):1215–21.
37. Shah K, Armamento-Villareal R, Parimi N, et al. Exercise training in obese older adults prevents increase in bone turnover and attenuates decrease in hip bone mineral density induced by weight loss despite decline in bone-active hormones. J Bone Miner Res 2011;26(12):2851–9.
38. Dube JJ, Amati F, Toledo FG, et al. Effects of weight loss and exercise on insulin resistance, and intramyocellular triacylglycerol, diacylglycerol and ceramide. Diabetologia 2011;54(5):1147–56.
39. Haus JM, Solomon TP, Lu L, et al. Intramyocellular lipid content and insulin sensitivity are increased following a short-term low-glycemic index diet and exercise intervention. Am J Physiol Endocrinol Metab 2011;301(3):E511–6.
40. Kelly KR, Haus JM, Solomon TP, et al. A low-glycemic index diet and exercise intervention reduces TNF (alpha) in isolated mononuclear cells of older, obese adults. J Nutr 2011;141(6):1089–94.
41. Santanasto AJ, Glynn NW, Newman MA, et al. Impact of weight loss on physical function with changes in strength, muscle mass, and muscle fat infiltration in overweight to moderately obese older adults: a randomized clinical trial. J Obes 2011; 2011 [pii:516576].
42. Chomentowski P, Dube JJ, Amati F, et al. Moderate exercise attenuates the loss of skeletal muscle mass that occurs with intentional caloric restriction-induced weight loss in older, overweight to obese adults. J Gerontol A Biol Sci Med Sci 2009;64(5):575–80.
43. Davidson LE, Hudson R, Kilpatrick K, et al. Effects of exercise modality on insulin resistance and functional limitation in older adults: a randomized controlled trial. Arch Intern Med 2009;169(2):122–31.
44. Lambert CP, Wright NR, Finck BN, et al. Exercise but not diet-induced weight loss decreases skeletal muscle inflammatory gene expression in frail obese elderly persons. J Appl Physiol 2008;105(2):473–8.
45. Solomon TP, Sistrun SN, Krishnan RK, et al. Exercise and diet enhance fat oxidation and reduce insulin resistance in older obese adults. J Appl Physiol 2008; 104(5):1313–9.
46. Villareal DT, Shah K, Banks MR, et al. Effect of weight loss and exercise therapy on bone metabolism and mass in obese older adults: a one-year randomized controlled trial. J Clin Endocrinol Metab 2008;93(6):2181–7.
47. Miller GD, Nicklas BJ, Davis C, et al. Intensive weight loss program improves physical function in older obese adults with knee osteoarthritis. Obesity (Silver Spring) 2006;14(7):1219–30.
48. Villareal DT, Banks M, Sinacore DR, et al. Effect of weight loss and exercise on frailty in obese older adults. Arch Intern Med 2006;166(8):860–6.
49. Messier SP, Loeser RF, Miller GD, et al. Exercise and dietary weight loss in overweight and obese older adults with knee osteoarthritis: the Arthritis, Diet, and Activity Promotion Trial. Arthritis Rheum 2004;50(5):1501–10.
50. Nicklas BJ, Ambrosius W, Messier SP, et al. Diet-induced weight loss, exercise, and chronic inflammation in older, obese adults: a randomized controlled clinical trial. Am J Clin Nutr 2004;79(4):544–51.

Protein and Older Persons

Juergen M. Bauer, MD, PhD*, Rebecca Diekmann, PhD

KEYWORDS

- Protein • Amino acids • Requirements • Supplementation • Older persons

KEY POINTS

- Older persons require more protein than their younger peers in order to maintain and build up muscle.
- Between 1.0 and 1.2 g protein per kilogram body weight should be consumed daily.
- The anabolic threshold for the daily protein and amino acid intake is higher in older than in younger adults, and should be set at approximately 25 to 30 g per meal, containing 2.5 to 2.8 g leucine.
- The source of protein and the amount of protein should be considered in all meals based on these recommendations for optimal protein intake.

INTRODUCTION

The percentage of older individuals more than 80 years of age is growing in all industrialized countries across the world, implying an increasing number of individuals who will be at risk of becoming dependent as a consequence of deteriorating strength and mobility. The optimization of protein intake is an important condition for preserving functionality and autonomy in older persons. Recent longitudinal studies provide evidence that the amount of protein consumed daily is associated with muscle mass, muscle strength, and physical function in older adults.[1,2]

FACTORS AFFECTING PROTEIN REQUIREMENTS IN OLDER AGE

Several mechanisms may lead to an insufficient protein intake in older people. In general, older people have decreasing energy needs, which is mainly a consequence of changes in physical activity. If the percentage of protein remains identical to that in the younger population, this decline in energy intake leads to an insufficient intake of protein. In older individuals, the requirement of protein should therefore always be calculated based on their BW. Age-associated anorexia, certain comorbidities, neurosensory changes in appetite and food preference, as well as bad dental status may be underlying reasons for a low intake of energy and, in parallel, of protein.

Department of Geriatric Medicine, Carl von Ossietzky Universität Oldenburg, Klinikum Oldenburg gGmbH, Rahel-Straus-Street 10, 26133 Oldenburg, Germany
* Corresponding author.
E-mail address: juergenmbauer@web.de

Clin Geriatr Med 31 (2015) 327–338
http://dx.doi.org/10.1016/j.cger.2015.04.002 **geriatric.theclinics.com**
0749-0690/15/$ – see front matter

Especially in older individuals with dental problems, preferences may shift toward foods that are rich in carbohydrates and fat and that have less protein.[3] The capacity to make use of the ingested protein anabolically may be reduced in older individuals by several pathomechanisms. The aging process is accompanied by an increasing anabolic resistance that affects muscle protein synthesis. This anabolic resistance is caused by numerous factors, such as decreased protein digestion and resorption as well as increased splanchnic sequestration of amino acids. In parallel, the postprandial availability of amino acids may be negatively affected by impaired muscle perfusion, which decreases the uptake of dietary amino acids by muscle.[4] In this context, an increase in insulin resistance with age may also be of relevance. In addition, certain subgroups of older persons have a greater need for protein because of their comorbidities (eg, inflammatory diseases). An overview of the mechanisms described earlier is provided in **Fig. 1**.[5]

At present, the World Health Organization, the US Institute of Medicine, and the European Safety Authority recommend a daily intake of 0.8 g/kg body weight (BW) for all adults, without any consideration of age.[6–8] These recommendations were based almost exclusively on nitrogen balance studies that, in most instances, included only a limited number of healthy older subjects, which is not representative of the older population in general. In the nitrogen balance studies a median estimated nitrogen requirement of 105 mg/kg BW per day was documented, which corresponds with 0.66 g of good-quality protein. The 97.5th percentile, 0.8 g protein/kg BW, was therefore set as the recommended daily allowance.[9] Nitrogen balance studies are based on the principle that protein constitutes the major source of nitrogen in the body. Therefore, loss of nitrogen represents a loss of protein. In nitrogen balance studies, nitrogen

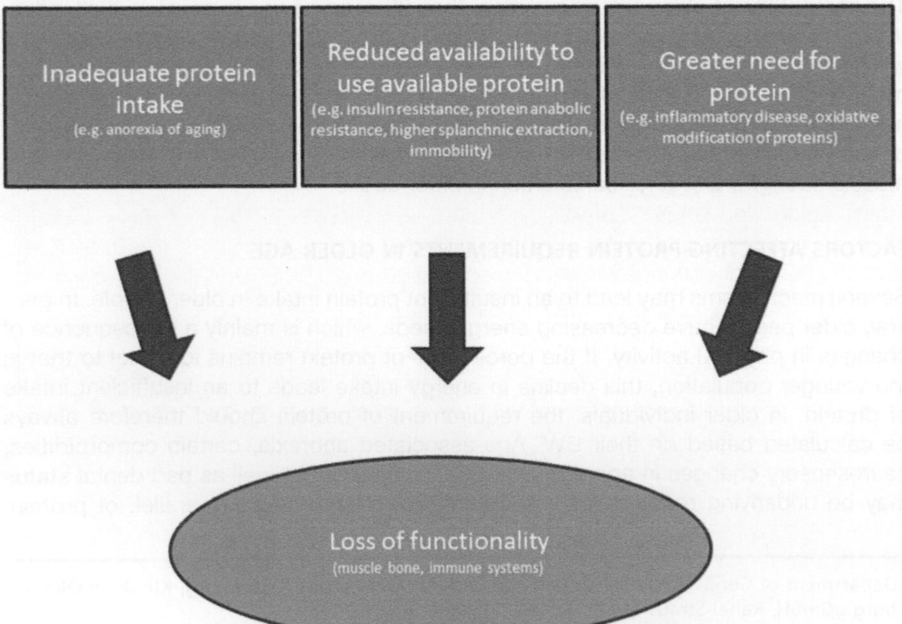

Fig. 1. Age-associated causes of protein deficits. (*From* Bauer J, Biolo G, Cederholm T, et al. Evidence-based recommendations for optimal dietary protein intake in older people: a position paper from the PROT-AGE Study Group. J Am Med Dir Assoc 2013;14(8):544; with permission.)

intake is documented well for a minimum of 5 days and a precise measurement of excreted nitrogen is taken. Because of this challenging method, few sources of error are present (eg, it is difficult to quantify all routes of nitrogen intake and loss).[5] Especially for older adults, who are represented to a very small extent in these studies, the age-associated changes in protein metabolism and altered requirements caused by comorbidities were considered insufficiently.

PROTEIN INTAKE IN OLDER PEOPLE

Protein Intake in Different Settings

Differences in protein intake between several settings have been documented in recent studies. In the general population, the intake of protein per kilogram BW decreases with age, as shown by Fulgoni[10] from NHANES (National Health and Nutrition Examination Survey) data from 2003/2004 (**Fig. 2**). From 5% to 6% of the population more than the age of 70 years consumed less than the estimated average requirement.[10] The German National Consumption Survey II identified 13.8% of older men and 15.2% of older women, both aged between 65 and 80 years, with a protein intake less than 0.8 g/kg BW/d.[11] Tieland and colleagues[12] observed a dependence of protein intake on functional status. Although community-dwelling older adults had an average intake of 1.1 g protein/kg BW, this amount decreased to 0.8 g protein/kg BW in nursing home residents. Ten percent of community-dwelling individuals and 35% of nursing home residents had an intake of less than 0.7 g protein/kg BW/d. A strong association between protein intake and cognitive as well as functional status was documented in a Finnish nursing home study by Vikstedt and colleagues.[13] Forty-seven percent of the residents consumed less than 60 g, and 11% less than 40 g, of protein per day. The oldest residents had the lowest consumption of protein.

Association with Muscle Mass, Muscle Strength, and Functionality

The benefit of higher protein intake in older persons has been documented in large epidemiologic and smaller clinical studies, showing an association between protein consumption and muscle mass as well as muscle strength.

Based on an analysis of the data of 2066 healthy adults who participated in the Health, Aging, and Body Composition Study, an association between protein intake and a decline in muscle mass during a follow-up period of 3 years was observed. Food frequency questionnaires were used to determine protein intake; muscle mass

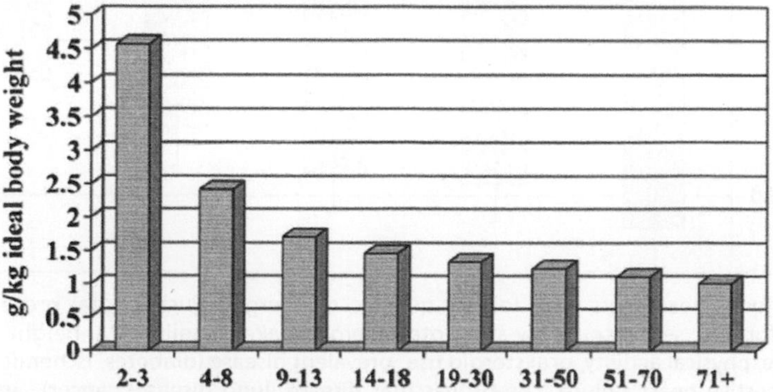

Fig. 2. Protein intake (grams per kilogram body weight). (*From* Fulgoni VL 3rd. Current protein intake in America: analysis of the National Health and Nutrition Examination Survey, 2003–2004. Am J Clin Nutr 2008;87(5):1556S; with permission.)

was measured by dual energy x-ray absorptiometry (DEXA). Subjects in the highest quintile of protein intake had a 40% lower loss of muscle mass than subjects in the lowest quintile (**Fig. 3**).[2] Consequently, a reduced protein intake led to increased muscle mass loss. This longitudinal observation provides evidence that low protein intake causes muscle loss in older adults.

In 2011, Campbell and colleagues[14] identified that a protein intake of 0.8 g/kg BW/d in a small group of seniors was associated with a reduction of muscle mass in the thigh over a period of 14 weeks, whereas body weight remained stable during this intervention. Gaillard and colleagues[15] measured a higher requirement for hospital patients than for healthy older people by using the nitrogen balance method.

Recently, the positive association between higher protein intake and improved performance was confirmed by data from the Women's Health and Aging study that covered a follow-up of almost 6 years.[16] In addition, Beasley and colleagues[17] were able to show in a very recent study that higher biomarker-calibrated protein intake was inversely associated with forearm fracture and, additionally, with better maintenance of total bone mineral density and bone mineral density of the hip. However, it was not possible to determine any association with total fracture or hip fracture. Biomarker-calibrated protein intake was calculated by using regression equations that were developed based on the Women's Health Initiative clinical trials and observational study Nutritional Biomarkers Study.[18]

RECENT CONSENSUS RECOMMENDATIONS FOR PROTEIN INTAKE IN OLDER PERSONS

Since 2013, 3 consensus articles on recommendations for protein intake in older adults have been published by international working groups. The contributing experts concluded that an optimal protein intake in this population should be higher than 0.8 g/kg BW/d. All working groups considered an amount of 1.0 to 1.2 g/kg BW/d as suitable for preserving functionality in healthy older adults.[5,19,20] The recommended intake would approximate 13% to 16% of total calories in most individuals, remaining within the macronutrient distribution range for protein (10%–35% of total calories). In

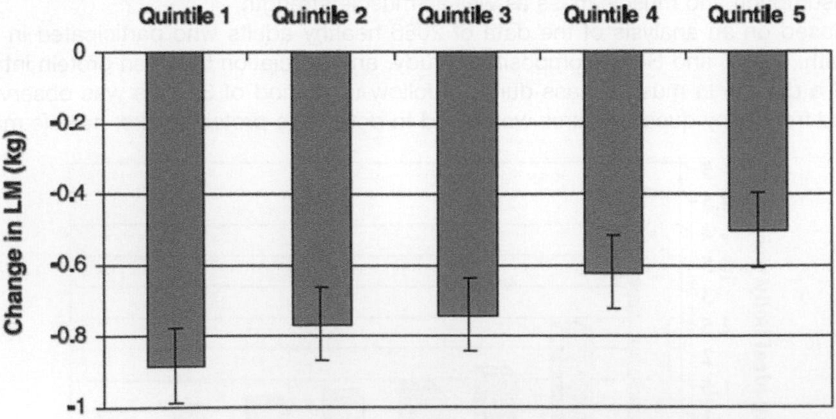

Fig. 3. Adjusted lean mass (LM) loss by quintile of energy-adjusted total protein intake. Adjusted for age, sex, race, study site, total energy intake, baseline LM, height, smoking, alcohol use, physical activity, oral steroid use, prevalent disease (diabetes, ischemic heart disease, congestive heart failure, cerebrovascular disease, lung disease, cancer), and interim hospitalizations. (*From* Houston DK, Nicklas BJ, Ding J, et al. Dietary protein intake is associated with lean mass change in older, community-dwelling adults: the Health, Aging, and Body Composition (Health ABC) Study. Am J Clin Nutr 2008;87(1):153; with permission.)

the presence of acute or chronic disease, protein intake may be increased up to 1.5 g/kg BW/d. If a protein intake of more than 1.2 g/kg BW/d is recommended, the satiating effect of protein must be considered, because it may interfere with the required intake of calories. An overview of current protein recommendations is presented in **Table 1**.

SUPPLEMENTATION

Several studies tested supplementation with protein and amino acids in older persons. They focused on different amounts of protein supplementation, on protein quality, and on the timing of supplementation.

Amount and Timing of Protein Intake

The timing and distribution of protein intake seem to play an important role in protein synthesis. Mamerow and colleagues[21] examined the 24-hour mixed muscle protein fractional synthesis rate with evenly distributed protein intake without carbohydrates at breakfast, lunch, and dinner against a skewed protein meal at dinner. They detected a 25% higher rate for the evenly distributed approach. Bollwein and colleagues[22] found

Table 1
Overview of current protein recommendations

	Institute of Medicine for Adults[a,7]	Recommendations by the PROT-AGE Study Group[b,5]	Recommendations by the ESPEN Group[19]	ESCEO Guidelines for Postmenopausal Women[20]
Healthy older adults	0.8 g/kg BW/d	1.0–1.2 g/kg BW/d 25–30 g protein/meal, including 2.5–2.8 g leucine	1.0–1.2 g/kg BW/d	50–71 y: 1.0 g/kg BW/d 71+ y: 1.0–1.2 g/kg BW/d 20–25 g protein/meal
Older adults with an acute or chronic illness	—	1.2–1.5 g/kg BW/d, adults with severe illness or injury or marked malnutrition need as much as 2.0 g/kg BW/d	1.2–1.5 g/kg BW/d; even higher when severely ill or malnourished	—
Physical activity	—	Endurance exercise at 30 min/d, include resistance training when possible, 2–3 per week for 10–15 min or more 20 g protein supplement after exercise	Daily physical activity (including resistance training) as long as possible	Regular physical activity/exercise 3–5 times/wk combined with protein intake in close proximity to exercise

Abbreviations: ESCEO, European Society for Clinical and Economic Aspects of Osteoporosis and Osteoarthritis; ESPEN, The European Society for Clinical Nutrition and Metabolism; PROT-AGE, International study group to review dietary protein needs with aging.
[a] Recommendations are regardless of gender and age for all adults.
[b] All adults older than 65 years are included, regardless of gender.
Data from Refs.[5,7,19,20]

a more uneven distribution of protein intake over the day in frail individuals with lower intake at breakfast and higher intake at lunch, whereas the median of the daily intake did not differ between robust prefrail and frail individuals. Even if these studies tend toward a recommendation of protein meals distributed evenly over the day, some studies have challenged this perspective and tested pulse feeding of protein.

For example, Bouillaine and colleagues[23] showed a significant increase in the lean mass index by providing protein pulse feeding compared with spread feeding in a group of 66 older patients in rehabilitation with malnutrition or a risk for malnutrition. Before a final conclusion can be drawn on this topic, both strategies (evenly distributed protein intake and pulse feeding) have to be tested in studies with extended intervention periods.

With regard to protein quality, branched-chain amino acids are highly relevant for the anabolic effect of protein. Leucine was identified as the most important branched-chain amino acid, which is why its effect in older individuals has been examined in several recent studies.

Lustgarten and colleagues[24] showed that 7 metabolites of branched-chain amino acids were associated with the muscle cross-sectional area and fat-free mass index in a cohort of 73 older persons with functional limitations.

Essential amino acid supplements were tested in intervention studies by several researchers. Ferrando and colleagues[25] provided a mix of all essential amino acids for 10 days versus placebo in a bed rest study, and found minor evidence for a better performance (eg, transfer time) in the intervention group. An increase in lean mass compared with baseline values was observed in a 3-month study with essential amino acids versus placebo.[26]

Based on their specific pattern of amino acids, including their percentage of leucine, proteins have been defined as fast and slow proteins. Fast proteins have a superior digestion rate, and are expected to show an additional anabolic effect on the protein balance. Whey protein may be considered as fast protein. Whey protein in fruit juice was tested versus fruit juice only by Björkmann and colleagues.[27] Protein supplementation resulted in a significant improvement in walking and toilet assistance after 6 months. Gryson and colleagues[28] showed that the leucine balance in older adults was improved to a larger degree with a high-protein diet (1.2 g/kg BW/d) compared with an adequate-protein diet (1.0 g/kg BW/d). This effect was strongest for soluble milk proteins, which are regarded as fast proteins. Tieland and colleagues[12] found an association between supplementation with milk protein and physical function. The intervention group, which received 15 g of milk protein for 24 weeks, showed a significantly higher Short Physical Performance Battery score than the control group.

The specific anabolic effects of leucine have been tested in several recent studies. In a small study by Wall and colleagues[29] involving 24 older adults, the effect of casein protein with or without 2.5 g of crystalline leucine on postprandial incorporation into muscle protein was tested. Postprandial muscle protein synthesis rates were improved with leucine coingestion. Three different doses of whey protein (10 g, 20 g, and 35 g) were tested to measure plasma peak values of marker amino acids, whole-body protein net balance, and postprandial muscle protein accretion in 48 older men. The best effect on all 3 outcome parameters was shown for the highest protein doses.[30]

According to the results discussed earlier, a higher intake of protein, especially those containing a high percentage of branched-chain amino acids, seems to create an additional anabolic benefit for protein synthesis. Because of its high amount of leucine and its characteristic as a fast protein, whey protein may be regarded as a suitable example. However, further evidence from extended longitudinal studies is required to verify the clinical relevance of supplementation with proteins that are fast and rich in leucine.

POSSIBLE CEILING EFFECT OF HIGHER PROTEIN INTAKE ON PROTEIN SYNTHESIS

A ceiling effect for a higher protein intake with regard to its positive effect on protein synthesis is discussed in recent publications. Walrand and colleagues[31] compared the effect of an increased protein intake on whole-body protein synthesis and muscle mitochondrial function in healthy younger adults versus older adults in a study involving 10 days of usual-protein (1.5 g protein/kg fat-free mass [FFM] per day) and high-protein (3.0 g protein/kg FFM per day) diets. Net daily nitrogen balance increased in both young and older subjects but, in parallel, the postabsorptive use of protein as fuel also increased. The investigators concluded that neither whole-body protein synthesis nor muscle mitochondrial function were affected positively by a short-term high-protein diet. Symons and colleagues[32] examined muscle protein synthesis by providing either a single moderate protein serving (30 g) or a large protein serving (90 g protein). They showed that an amount exceeding 30 g protein per meal failed to enhance muscle protein synthesis further. This effect was observed in both younger and older subjects.

In contrast, Deutz and Wolfe[33] measured net protein synthesis by calculating the difference between the rate of synthesis and the rate of breakdown. They concluded that there is no upper limit for the anabolic response to increasing amounts of protein during a meal. Although protein synthesis shows a ceiling effect with higher protein intake, this is not the case for the associated decrease in protein breakdown.

RELEVANCE OF PROTEIN INTAKE FOR OLDER PATIENTS

Hip Fracture and Knee Arthroplasty

According to recent studies, prevalence of malnutrition in patients with hip fractures ranges from 30% to more than 50%.[34,35] Malnutrition in general, and especially protein deficiency, has to be regarded as a predisposing factor for osteoporosis and sarcopenia, which are both key factors in the causes of fall-related fractures. Although protein deficiency is present in many patients with hip fracture at hospital admission, it may deteriorate further as a consequence of insufficient protein intake during the hospital stay. Protein supplementation may therefore be considered to be highly relevant in this patient population, which is at a very high risk of experiencing a rapid and persistent functional decline.

The supplementation of 18 to 24 g of protein and 500 kcal per day versus a standard hospital diet was tested in 126 older patients with hip fractures. Significant positive effects were observed with regard to body mass index, length of stay, and number of infections.[36]

Botella-Carretero and colleagues[37] tested whether supplementation with 40 g of protein plus 400 kcal was beneficial for patients with hip fractures during their hospital stays. Compared with the control group, significantly fewer postoperative complications were found in the intervention group. Supplementation with 20 g of protein versus an isocaloric placebo was tested in a cohort of 82 patients with osteoporotic hip fractures. On average, patients receiving the protein supplementation required a significantly shorter stay in rehabilitation hospitals.[38]

Two systematic reviews from 2009 and 2010 showed that supplementation benefited patients with hip fractures with regard to a reduced risk of complications and a shorter rehabilitation time.[39,40] However, the need for additional well-conducted intervention studies was established in both articles.

During rehabilitation, the combined effect of physical exercise and protein supplementation may be beneficial in patients with hip fractures.[41] In this context, the ingestion of protein supplements in temporal proximity to physical exercise should be advised.

Dreyer and colleagues[42] focused on patients with total knee arthroplasty and the subsequent atrophy of muscle. They tested the effect of 20 g of essential amino acids twice a day from 1 week before until 2 weeks after surgery in a treatment group versus a placebo group. In the supplemented group, quadriceps muscle atrophy was significantly lower, and resulted in better mobility tests 2 and 6 weeks after surgery. All patients had bilateral MRI of the lower extremities between the anterior superior iliac spine and the tibia plateau 2 weeks before surgery and 6 weeks after surgery.

Osteoporosis

The association between bone mineral density (BMD) and protein intake was described in several cross-sectional and longitudinal studies. In a cross-sectional study that included 1077 women, protein intake was estimated by food frequency questionnaires, and hip BMD was measured by DEXA. Subjects in the lowest tertile of protein consumption (<66 g/d) had significantly lower hip BMD than subjects in the highest tertile of protein consumption (>87 g/d).[43] Meng and colleagues[44] investigated the relationship between protein intake and bone mineral content (BMC) in a longitudinal study. Protein intake at baseline was assessed by food frequency questionnaires. At 5 years, BMC was measured by DEXA. Positive associations were found between baseline protein intake and BMC. In a smaller study with 33 subjects, the effects of supplementation with lower and higher amounts of protein over 9 weeks on biochemical markers of bone turnover were investigated. Higher protein consumption was associated with higher insulinlike growth factor-I levels, a biomarker for bone growth, and lower levels of urinary N-telopeptide, a marker for bone resorption.[45] In a systematic review from 2009, including 61 trials, the positive effect of an increased protein intake on BMD was documented.[40]

Summarizing the available evidence, a higher protein intake of 1.0 g/kg BW per day can be recommended with regard to its positive effects on bone health.

Protein Intake and Chronic Kidney Disease

The functional capacity of the kidney decreases in most individuals with increasing age. Evidence of a higher protein intake posing a risk to kidney function may be regarded as inconclusive. In a 5-year observational study including women more than 60 years of age, no deterioration of the glomerular filtration rate (GFR) was observed, whereas protein intake was documented with a mean of 1.1 g/kg BW/d.[46] In contrast, in the Nurses' Health Study, higher protein consumption was associated with decreasing GFR in women with initial mild renal failure.[47]

In 2013, the International Society of Renal Nutrition and Metabolism published recommendations for adults with chronic renal failure, including those on dialysis. People with renal failure showed high needs of energy, of around 30 to 35 kcal/kg BW/d. A protein intake of 0.6 to 0.8 g/kg BW/d has been recommended for persons with chronic kidney disease who are not on dialysis. These recommendations should be adapted toward 1.0 g/kg BW per day in individuals with disease or injury, especially if a patient with chronic kidney disease shows signs of sarcopenia. Older adults on peritoneal dialysis or on hemodialysis should consume more than 1.2 g/kg BW per day to be able to compensate for the catabolic effect of dialysis.[48] This amount may be increased up to 1.5 g/kg BW per day, if feasible. In parallel, an adequate intake of energy has to be achieved. An overview is presented in **Table 2**.

Table 2
Recommended protein intakes for patients with CKD

Nondialysis CKD		Hemodialysis	Peritoneal Dialysis
PROT-ACE recommendations for older people with kidney disease	Severe CKD, GFR<30[a]: limit protein intake to 0.8 g/kg BW[b]/d Moderate CKD, 30<GFR<60: protein >0.8 g/kg BW[b]/d is safe, but GFR should be monitored twice a year Mild CKD, GFR>60: increase protein intake per patient needs	>1.2 g/kg BW[b]/d or, if achievable, 1.5 g/kg BW[b]/d[c]	>1.2 g/kg BW[b]/d or, if achievable, 1.5 g/kg BW[b]/d[c]

Abbreviation: CKD, chronic kidney disease.
[a] GFR is measured in mL/min/1.73 m^2.
[b] Recommendations are based on ideal BW. Regular follow-up supports compliance.
[c] Prospective studies targeting these high protein intakes in older patients on hemodialysis/peritoneal dialysis are not available.
From Bauer J, Biolo G, Cederholm T, et al. Evidence-based recommendations for optimal dietary protein intake in older people: a position paper from the PROT-AGE Study Group. J Am Med Dir Assoc 2013;14(8):542–59; with permission.

SUMMARY

Current evidence supports the recommendation of a higher protein intake than 0.8 g/kg BW per day in older persons, because it contributes to stabilizing functionality and increasing the potential for successful aging. Individual recommendations have to take into account relevant comorbidities, including kidney function. The additional benefit of specified amino acid mixtures has to be documented in adequately sized intervention studies. However, preliminary evidence in this direction seems to be promising. Nutritional measures including protein supplementation are highly relevant for the preservation and improvement of physical function in older persons. However, in most cases they should be part of a multifaceted program that includes physical exercise. Nonetheless, some patients are unable to exercise adequately; for example, temporarily after certain orthopedic operations. In this case, sole protein supplementation may be highly relevant.

REFERENCES

1. Beasley JM, LaCroix AZ, Neuhouser ML, et al. Protein intake and incident frailty in the Women's Health Initiative observational study. J Am Geriatr Soc 2010;58(6): 1063–71.
2. Houston DK, Nicklas BJ, Ding J, et al. Dietary protein intake is associated with lean mass change in older, community-dwelling adults: the Health, Aging, and Body Composition (Health ABC) Study. Am J Clin Nutr 2008;87(1):150–5.
3. Volpi E, Campbell WW, Dwyer JT, et al. Is the optimal level of protein intake for older adults greater than the recommended dietary allowance? J Gerontol A Biol Sci Med Sci 2013;68(6):677–81.

4. Burd NA, Gorissen SH, van Loon LJ. Anabolic resistance of muscle protein synthesis with aging. Exerc Sport Sci Rev 2013;41(3):169–73.
5. Bauer J, Biolo G, Cederholm T, et al. Evidence-based recommendations for optimal dietary protein intake in older people: a position paper from the PROT-AGE study group. J Am Med Dir Assoc 2013;14(8):542–59.
6. World Health Organization. Protein and amino acid requirements in human nutrition: report of a joint WHO/FAO/UNU Expert Consultation. Geneva, Switzerland: WHO Press; 2007 (Report 935).
7. Dietary reference intakes for energy, carbohydrate, fiber, fat, fatty acids, cholesterol, protein, and amino acids - Institute of Medicine. Available at: http://www.iom.edu/Reports/2002/Dietary-Reference-Intakes-for-Energy-Carbohydrate-Fiber-Fat-Fatty-Acids-Cholesterol-Protein-and-Amino-Acids.aspx. Accessed December 16, 2014.
8. European Safety Authority. Scientific opinion dietary reference values for protein. EFSA J 2012;(10):2557. Available at: http://www.efsa.europa.eu/en/search/doc/2557.pdf. Accessed December 16, 2014.
9. Bauer JM, Diekmann R. Protein supplementation with aging. Curr Opin Clin Nutr Metab Care 2015;18(1):24–31.
10. Fulgoni VL 3rd. Current protein intake in America: analysis of the National Health and Nutrition Examination Survey, 2003-2004. Am J Clin Nutr 2008;87(5):1554S–7S.
11. Max Rubner-Institut MRI, Bundesforschungsinstitut für Ernährung und Lebensmittel. Ergebnisbericht Teil 2 Nationale Verzehrsstudie II. 2008. Available at: http://www.mri.bund.de/fileadmin/Institute/EV/NVSII_Abschlussbericht_Teil_2.pdf. Accessed February 13, 2015.
12. Tieland M, van de Rest O, Dirks ML, et al. Protein supplementation improves physical performance in frail elderly people: a randomized, double-blind, placebo-controlled trial. J Am Med Dir Assoc 2012;13(8):720–6.
13. Vikstedt T, Suominen MH, Joki A, et al. Nutritional status, energy, protein, and micronutrient intake of older service house residents. J Am Med Dir Assoc 2011; 12(4):302–7.
14. Campbell WW, Trappe TA, Wolfe RR, et al. The recommended dietary allowance for protein may not be adequate for older people to maintain skeletal muscle. J Gerontol A Biol Sci Med Sci 2001;56(6):M373–80.
15. Gaillard C, Alix E, Boirie Y, et al. Are elderly hospitalized patients getting enough protein? J Am Geriatr Soc 2008;56(6):1045–9.
16. Beasley JM, Wertheim BC, LaCroix AZ, et al. Biomarker-calibrated protein intake and physical function in the Women's Health Initiative. J Am Geriatr Soc 2013; 61(11):1863–71.
17. Beasley JM, LaCroix AZ, Larson JC, et al. Biomarker-calibrated protein intake and bone health in the Women's Health Initiative clinical trials and observational study. Am J Clin Nutr 2014;99(4):934–40.
18. Neuhouser ML, Tinker L, Shaw PA, et al. Use of recovery biomarkers to calibrate nutrient consumption self-reports in the Women's Health Initiative. Am J Epidemiol 2008;167(10):1247–59.
19. Deutz NE, Bauer JM, Barazzoni R, et al. Protein intake and exercise for optimal muscle function with aging: recommendations from the ESPEN Expert Group. Clin Nutr 2014;33(6):929–36.
20. Rizzoli R, Stevenson JC, Bauer JM, et al. The role of dietary protein and vitamin D in maintaining musculoskeletal health in postmenopausal women: a consensus statement from the European Society for Clinical and Economic Aspects of Osteoporosis and Osteoarthritis (ESCEO). Maturitas 2014;79(1):122–32.

21. Mamerow MM, Mettler JA, English KL, et al. Dietary protein distribution positively influences 24-h muscle protein synthesis in healthy adults. J Nutr 2014;144(6):876–80.
22. Bollwein J, Diekmann R, Kaiser MJ, et al. Distribution but not amount of protein intake is associated with frailty: a cross-sectional investigation in the region of Nurnberg. Nutr J 2013;12(1):109.
23. Bouillanne O, Curis E, Hamon-Vilcot B, et al. Impact of protein pulse feeding on lean mass in malnourished and at-risk hospitalized elderly patients: a randomized controlled trial. Clin Nutr 2013;32(2):186–92.
24. Lustgarten MS, Price LL, Chale A, et al. Branched chain amino acids are associated with muscle mass in functionally limited older adults. J Gerontol A Biol Sci Med Sci 2014;69(6):717–24.
25. Ferrando AA, Paddon-Jones D, Hays NP, et al. EAA supplementation to increase nitrogen intake improves muscle function during bed rest in the elderly. Clin Nutr 2010;29(1):18–23.
26. Dillon EL, Sheffield-Moore M, Paddon-Jones D, et al. Amino acid supplementation increases lean body mass, basal muscle protein synthesis, and insulin-like growth factor-I expression in older women. J Clin Endocrinol Metab 2009;94(5):1630–7.
27. Björkman M, Finne-Soveri H, Tilvis R. Whey protein supplementation in nursing home residents. A randomized controlled trial. Eur Geriatr Med 2012;3(3):161–6. Available at: http://www.europeangeriaticmedicine.com/article/S1878-7649(12)00073-3/references. Accessed March 2, 2015.
28. Gryson C, Walrand S, Giraudet C, et al. "Fast proteins" with a unique essential amino acid content as an optimal nutrition in the elderly: growing evidence. Clin Nutr 2014;33(4):642–8.
29. Wall BT, Hamer HM, de Lange A, et al. Leucine co-ingestion improves post-prandial muscle protein accretion in elderly men. Clin Nutr 2013;32(3):412–9.
30. Pennings B, Boirie Y, Senden JM, et al. Whey protein stimulates postprandial muscle protein accretion more effectively than do casein and casein hydrolysate in older men. Am J Clin Nutr 2011;93(5):997–1005.
31. Walrand S, Short KR, Bigelow ML, et al. Functional impact of high protein intake on healthy elderly people. Am J Physiol Endocrinol Metab 2008;295(4):E921–8.
32. Symons TB, Sheffield-Moore M, Wolfe RR, et al. A moderate serving of high-quality protein maximally stimulates skeletal muscle protein synthesis in young and elderly subjects. J Am Diet Assoc 2009;109(9):1582–6.
33. Deutz NE, Wolfe RR. Is there a maximal anabolic response to protein intake with a meal? Clin Nutr 2013;32(2):309–13.
34. Drevet S, Bioteau C, Maziere S, et al. Prevalence of protein-energy malnutrition in hospital patients over 75 years of age admitted for hip fracture. Orthop Traumatol Surg Res 2014;100(6):669–74.
35. Bell J, Bauer J, Capra S, et al. Barriers to nutritional intake in patients with acute hip fracture: time to treat malnutrition as a disease and food as a medicine? Can J Physiol Pharmacol 2013;91(6):489–95.
36. Myint MW, Wu J, Wong E, et al. Clinical benefits of oral nutritional supplementation for elderly hip fracture patients: a single blind randomised controlled trial. Age Ageing 2013;42(1):39–45.
37. Botella-Carretero JI, Iglesias B, Balsa JA, et al. Perioperative oral nutritional supplements in normally or mildly undernourished geriatric patients submitted to surgery for hip fracture: a randomized clinical trial. Clin Nutr 2010;29(5):574–9.

38. Schurch MA, Rizzoli R, Slosman D, et al. Protein supplements increase serum insulin-like growth factor-I levels and attenuate proximal femur bone loss in patients with recent hip fracture. A randomized, double-blind, placebo-controlled trial. Ann Intern Med 1998;128(10):801–9.
39. Avenell A, Handoll HH. Nutritional supplementation for hip fracture aftercare in older people. Cochrane Database Syst Rev 2010;(1):CD001880.
40. Milne AC, Potter J, Vivanti A, et al. Protein and energy supplementation in elderly people at risk from malnutrition. Cochrane Database Syst Rev 2009;(2):CD003288.
41. Fiatarone Singh MA. Exercise, nutrition and managing hip fracture in older persons. Curr Opin Clin Nutr Metab Care 2014;17(1):12–24.
42. Dreyer HC, Strycker LA, Senesac HA, et al. Essential amino acid supplementation in patients following total knee arthroplasty. J Clin Invest 2013;123(11): 4654–66.
43. Devine A, Dick IM, Islam AF, et al. Protein consumption is an important predictor of lower limb bone mass in elderly women. Am J Clin Nutr 2005;81(6):1423–8.
44. Meng X, Zhu K, Devine A, et al. A 5-year cohort study of the effects of high protein intake on lean mass and BMC in elderly postmenopausal women. J Bone Miner Res 2009;24(11):1827–34.
45. Dawson-Hughes B, Harris SS, Rasmussen H, et al. Effect of dietary protein supplements on calcium excretion in healthy older men and women. J Clin Endocrinol Metab 2004;89(3):1169–73.
46. Beasley JM, Aragaki AK, LaCroix AZ, et al. Higher biomarker-calibrated protein intake is not associated with impaired renal function in postmenopausal women. J Nutr 2011;141(8):1502–7.
47. Knight EL, Stampfer MJ, Hankinson SE, et al. The impact of protein intake on renal function decline in women with normal renal function or mild renal insufficiency. Ann Intern Med 2003;138(6):460–7.
48. Ikizler TA, Cano NJ, Franch H, et al. Prevention and treatment of protein energy wasting in chronic kidney disease patients: a consensus statement by the International Society of Renal Nutrition and Metabolism. Kidney Int 2013;84(6): 1096–107.

Gastric Emptying in the Elderly

Stijn Soenen, PhD*, Chris K. Rayner, MBBS, PhD, FRACP,
Michael Horowitz, MBBS, PhD, FRACP, Karen L. Jones, Dip App Sci, PhD

KEYWORDS

- Gastric emptying • Migrating motor complex • Neural and humoral feedback
- Scintigraphy • Breath tests • Ultrasonography • Glycemia • Blood pressure

KEY POINTS

- The gastric and small intestinal motor and humoral mechanisms responsible for normal gastric emptying in humans are complex and highly variable.
- Healthy aging seems associated with modest slowing of gastric emptying, but emptying generally remains within the normal range for young subjects.
- Parkinson disease and diabetes are examples of comorbidities that increase with advancing age and frequently have an impact on gastric emptying.
- The effects of aging on gastric emptying/motility are of relevance to the absorption kinetics of oral medications as well as the regulation of appetite, postprandial glycemia, and blood pressure.

INTRODUCTION

This article reviews the impact of healthy aging on gastric emptying, related motor and sensory function of the upper gut, and what is known about the underlying causes of disordered gastric emptying and their clinical significance. The techniques that may be used to measure gastric emptying also are addressed. The effects of aging on gastric emptying are of potential relevance to the absorption of oral medications as well as the regulation of appetite, postprandial glycemia, and blood pressure. Aging is associated with an increased prevalence of several diseases associated with abnormal, in particular delayed, gastric emptying.

Potential Competing Interests: None of the authors has any conflicts of interest to declare.
Sources of Support: S. Soenen was supported by a Royal Adelaide Hospital Mary Overton Early Career Research Fellowship and K.L. Jones by an NHMRC Senior Clinical Career Development Award (627011).
Discipline of Medicine, National Health and Medical Research Council of Australia (NHMRC) Centre of Research Excellence in Translating Nutritional Science to Good Health, Royal Adelaide Hospital, The University of Adelaide, Frome Road, Adelaide, South Australia 5000, Australia
* Corresponding author.
E-mail address: stijn.soenen@adelaide.edu.au

http://dx.doi.org/10.1016/j.cger.2015.04.003

MECHANISMS CONTROLLING GASTRIC EMPTYING

Gastric emptying reflects the coordinated motor activity of the proximal stomach, distal stomach (antrum and pylorus), and duodenum, which is controlled primarily by feedback from neural and humoral signals generated by the interaction of nutrients with the small intestine. The gastric and small intestinal mechanisms responsible for normal gastric emptying in humans are complex and highly variable: ingested food must be stored, mixed with digestive enzymes, ground into small particles, and delivered as a liquefied form to the duodenum at a rate that allows efficient digestion and absorption.

The Migrating Motor Complex

The synchronous periodic pattern of gastric motor activity during interdigestive/fasting periods, which moves from the stomach to the terminal ileum over a period of 90 to 120 minutes and is controlled by complex neurohumoral mechanisms, is called the migrating motor complex and comprises 4 phases.[1] This housekeeping complex generates peristaltic waves of activity and promotes passage of indigestible food products, cellular debris, and bacteria through the gastrointestinal tract. Phase I of the migrating motor complex is associated with motor quiescence with no contractions and lasts approximately 40 minutes; phase II is characterized by random contractions and lasts approximately 50 minutes (**Fig. 1**); and phase III is characterized by regular contractions with maximal amplitude for approximately 5 to 10 minutes (**Fig. 2**), followed by phase IV, a rapid decrease of the contractions, which may be absent or very short and, therefore, undetectable.

The migrating motor complex has a circadian pattern with reduced propagation velocity and shorter duration, particularly of phase II, at night. Contractions of the stomach are linked to an underlying electrical rhythm, generated by gastric pacemaker cells. These interstitial cells of Cajal are situated within the Auerbach plexus where they generate contractions within the antrum and pylorus at a rate of approximately 3 cycles per minute.[2] The muscular contractions are promoted by mediators, such

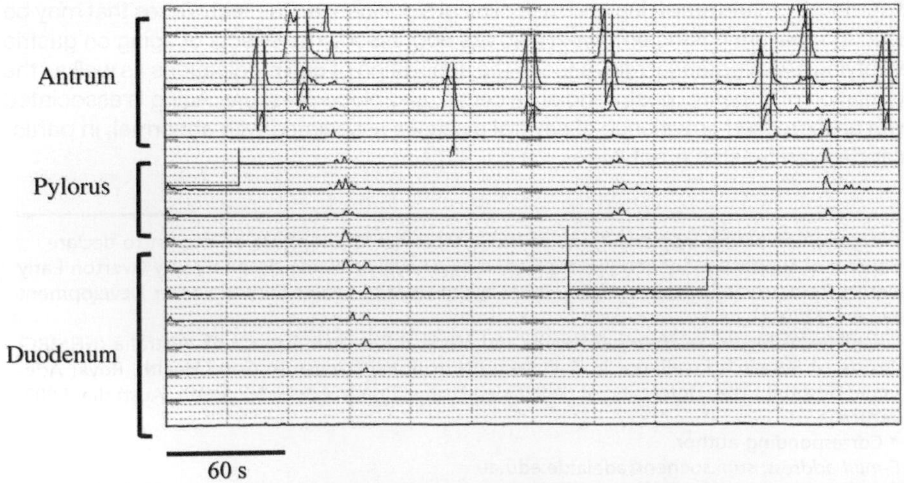

Fig. 1. Manometry recording during fasting conditions of irregular contractions of the migrating motor complex phase II, usually lasting approximately 50 minutes, using a 16-channel catheter for the assessment of pressures in the antropyloroduodenal region.

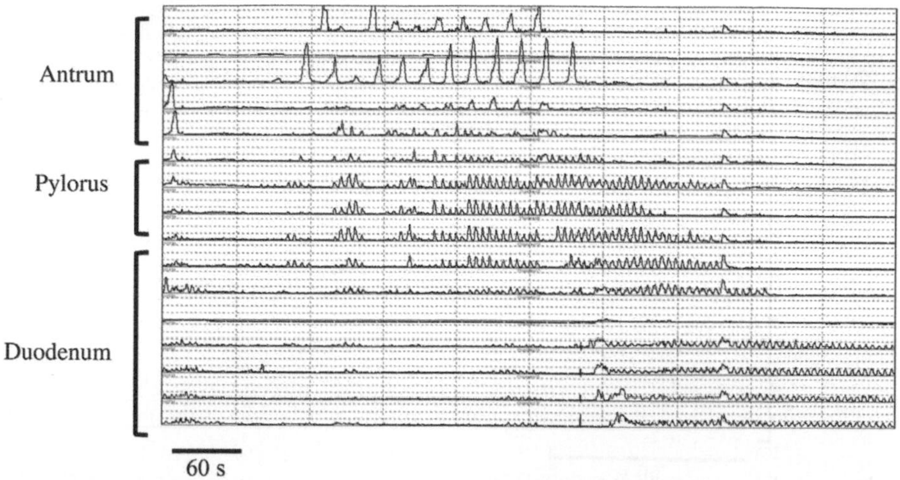

Fig. 2. Manometry recording during fasting conditions of regular contractions of the migrating motor complex phase III during which large indigestible solids are emptied from the stomach, usually lasting approximately 5 to 10 minutes, using a 16-channel catheter for the assessment of pressures in the antropyloroduodenal region.

as acetylcholine and the neuropeptide substance P, and inhibited by the vasoactive intestinal peptide, carbon monoxide, and nitric oxide.[3] Plasma concentrations of the hormone motilin, which is secreted from the duodenum and jejunum and in the myenteric plexus, are related to the pattern of the migrating motor complex, with peak concentrations at the start of phase III and lowest concentrations during phase I. Gastric pH fluctuates during the migrating motor complex, with the antral pH lowest at the start of phase III and highest at the start of phase I.

Motor Activity of the Stomach

Slowing of gastric emptying of nutrients occurs as a result of increased phasic and tonic pyloric pressure waves, acting as a resistance to outflow, and reductions in antral and proximal duodenal pressure waves (**Fig. 3**) as well as fundic tone and intragastric redistribution from the distal to the proximal stomach.[4–6] The integration of these mechanisms accounts for fine-tuning of pulsatile gastric outflow.

The proximal region of the stomach, comprising the fundus and much of the gastric body, undergoes an initial receptive relaxation and a subsequent prolonged adaptive relaxation and acts as a reservoir for the solid components of the meal while liquids begin to empty. Gastric compliance and accommodation, therefore, play an important part in the physiology of gastric emptying. The distal stomach is responsible for grinding solids into particles by irregular antral and pyloric contractions and for generating flow across the pylorus—the latter is predominantly pulsatile rather than continuous.[7,8] Transpyloric flow is bidirectional, so that both antegrade and retrograde flow occurs.[9–11] The characteristics of flow pulses (pulse, frequency, and volume) are subject to considerable variation reflecting changes in intragastric volume and small intestinal feedback. Tonic contraction of the proximal stomach also generates a pressure gradient, which facilitates gastric emptying.

Rate and Patterns of Gastric Emptying

As a result of the closely related motor functions of the stomach and small intestine, the rate of the energy delivery to the small intestine is relatively constant within an

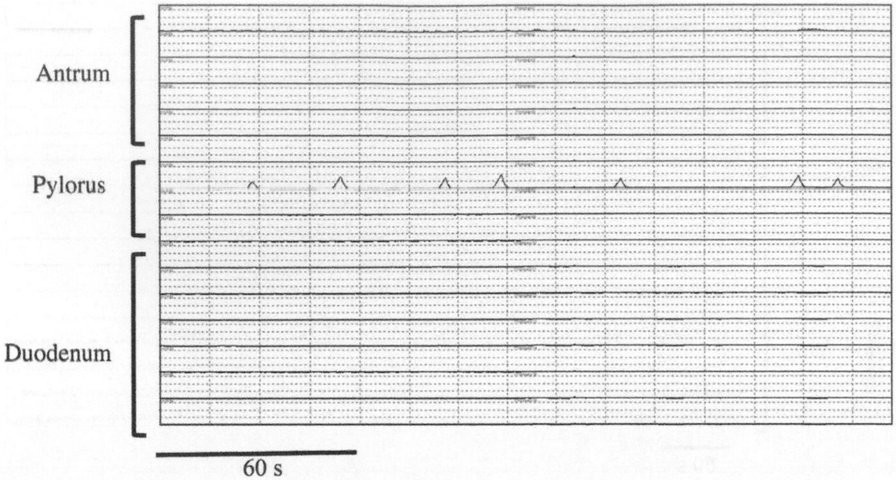

Fig. 3. Manometry recording during intraduodenal nutrient infusion of isolated pyloric pressure waves, defined as pyloric pressure waves that occur in the absence of pressure waves on adjacent antral and duodenal channels, using a 16-channel catheter for the assessment of pressures in the antropyloroduodenal region.

individual. In healthy individuals, the stomach usually empties at an overall rate of 1 to 4 kcal/min.[4,7,12] This substantial interindividual variation in the rate of gastric emptying contrasts with the modest intraindividual variation.[13] Gastric emptying of both solids and liquids may be slightly slower in pre- and postmenopausal women compared with men,[14] possibly reflecting differences in autonomic tone.[15] The rate of gastric emptying depends on meal composition (ie, liquids and/or solids and macronutrient content [proteins, carbohydrates, and fats]).[2,4]

There are major differences in patterns of gastric emptying of digestible and nondigestible solids and caloric and noncaloric liquids. Gastric emptying of digestible solids is characterized by a lag phase, before emptying commences, followed by an emptying phase that approximates a linear pattern, at least for the majority of emptying.[16] The lag phase (usually 20–40 min in duration) reflects the time taken for redistribution of food from the proximal to the distal stomach and for grinding of solid food into small particles with a diameter of less than 1 to 2 mm—a major rate-limiting step in gastric emptying of solids. Nondigestible solids (>5 mm) in size are emptied predominantly during phase III of the migrating motor complex (ie during interdigestive periods when high-amplitude antropyloric pressure waves produce sequential lumen occlusion in the proximal antrum).[17] In contrast to solids, volume and gravity are important driving forces in gastric emptying of noncaloric, isotonic liquids, which empty much faster than solids and in a nonlinear, overall monoexponential, pattern. Accordingly, gastric emptying of noncaloric isotonic liquids is affected by posture.[18] Caloric and hyperosmotic liquids empty from the stomach more slowly than noncaloric liquids and, after a variable, more rapid initial emptying phase, at an overall linear rate in response to the inhibitory feedback from small intestinal luminal receptors. Gastric emptying of caloric liquids is influenced by the presence of solid food in the stomach and gastric emptying of solids is modified by the presence of nutrient liquids.[19] After ingestion of a solid-liquid meal, the stomach retains solid food predominantly in the proximal stomach, until the majority (approximately 80%) of the liquid has emptied.

Intrinsic and Extrinsic Signals to Control Gastric Emptying

Patterns of motor activity, involving the circular and longitudinal layers of smooth muscle, which drive the emptying of the content of the stomach, extend throughout the length of the gut and are coordinated by plexuses of nerves within the gut wall known collectively as the enteric nervous system. Located in the submucosa (submucous plexus, which is involved in secretion and absorption and also motor control) and between the muscle layers (myenteric plexus, which is involved with initiation and control of smooth muscle contraction), this network contains a comparable number of neurons (approximately 100 million) to that present in the spinal cord.[20] The intrinsic sensory neurons, interneurons, and motor neurons that comprise the enteric nervous system control basic contractile activity, such as reflex responses to distension. These intrinsic patterns of gut motility are modulated by both extrinsic neural and humoral signals.

Central modulation of gut motility occurs via extrinsic sympathetic and parasympathetic nerves, whereas gut sensation is conveyed to higher centers by both the vagus and spinal afferent nerves, with noxious signals transmitted predominantly via the latter. Descending pathways to the spinal cord modulate the transmission of sensory signals.

Small intestinal mechanisms are highly sensitive to the presence of ingested nutrients.[21] The delivery of small amounts of nutrients directly into the small intestine has the capacity to slow gastric emptying by suppressing antral motility and increasing pyloric motility and fundic relaxation, mediated, at least in part, by the stimulation of gut hormone secretion (ie, cholecystokinin [CCK], glucagon-like peptide 1 [GLP-1], peptide tyrosine tyrosine [PYY], and gastric inhibitory peptide [GIP]).[22] Although circulating levels of motilin and ghrelin peak during fasting and are suppressed postprandially, these peptides also may influence gastric emptying.[23]

MEASUREMENT OF GASTRIC EMPTYING

The techniques that may be used to evaluate gastric emptying/motility are summarized in **Box 1**. Scintigraphy remains the gold standard for measurement of gastric emptying, and the use of dual isotopes allows both the solid and liquid components of a meal to be

Box 1
Techniques to evaluate gastric emptying/motility

Scintigraphy

Breath tests

Ultrasonography

Radiology (liquid barium sulfate, radio-opaque markers)

Applied potential tomography/epigastric impedance

Paracetamol absorption

Intubation and aspiration of gastric contents

CT scanning

MRI

High-resolution manometry

Electrogastrography

quantified.[24,25] Regional meal distribution can also be evaluated by defining regions of interest within the stomach.[5] Scintigraphy necessitates access to a gamma camera and is associated with radiation exposure and is, therefore, contraindicated in pregnancy and relatively contraindicated in children. Despite the long-term adoption of scintigraphy as a diagnostic tool, there remains a lack of standardization of the technique (eg, meal composition and volume, posture of subjects, frequency and duration of data acquisition, and parameters used to quantify gastric emptying).[26]

Breath tests represent an alternative approach, particularly when scintigraphy is not feasible,[2,24,26] and are based on the incorporation of Carbon-13-labeled substrates, usually Carbon-13-octanoic acid, into solid meals or nutrient liquid. The stable Carbon-13-isotope is emptied from the stomach and transported to the liver via the portal vein, where it is oxidized to $^{13}CO_2$. End-tidal breath samples are collected and Carbon-13 content measured using isotope ratio mass spectrometry; estimation of gastric emptying is obtained with mathematical modeling. The technique is noninvasive and does not expose patients to radiation and, therefore, is an option in pregnant or lactating women and in children. Furthermore, breath tests are cheaper than scintigraphy and, because samples can be sent to a central laboratory, may be undertaken in an office-based setting as well as in patients who cannot be easily transported within the hospital setting. Breath testing assumes normal small intestinal, hepatic, and pulmonary function, and testing in populations outside this range (eg, those with small intestinal malabsorption or pulmonary or liver disease) may be inaccurate. Breath testing has not been validated well in patients with markedly delayed gastric emptying; moreover, the gastric emptying rates are best regarded as notional, rather than accurate, unlike scintigraphy.

Ultrasonography is alternative method of measuring gastric emptying—its use is usually restricted to liquid or semisolid meals (**Fig. 4**).[22,27] Ultrasonography can be undertaken using a 2-D or 3-D technique. Measurements of antral area are used to derive gastric emptying in 2-D; the 3-D technique is more accurate compared with 2-D but requires additional equipment and expertise.[28,29] Advantages of this noninvasive technique include lack of radiation exposure and information on intragastric meal distribution and volume. The technique is operator dependent and more difficult in obesity.[24–26]

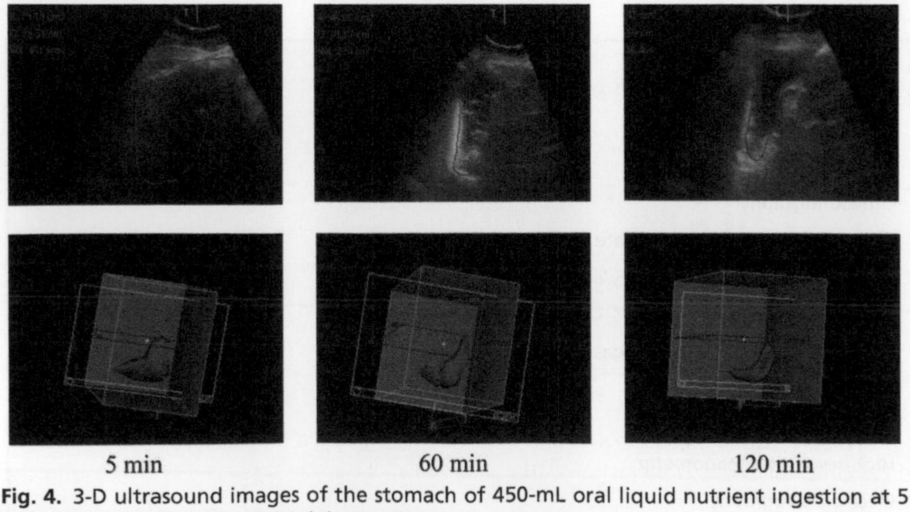

Fig. 4. 3-D ultrasound images of the stomach of 450-mL oral liquid nutrient ingestion at 5 (*left*), 60 (*center*), and 120 (*right*) minutes.

High-resolution manometry is used predominantly for research purposes to record the frequency, amplitude, and organization of lumen-occlusive contractions in the antrum, pylorus, and duodenum using a multilumen catheter with an array of side holes and/or a pyloric sleeve sensor.[30]

Proximal gastric relaxation in response to a meal can be evaluated in a laboratory using an electronic barostat; the volume of air required to maintain a fixed pressure in an intragastric bag is used as an index of proximal gastric tone.[31]

EFFECTS OF HEALTHY AGING ON GASTRIC EMPTYING AND MOTILITY

It is well recognized that aging is characterized by a diminished homeostatic regulation of many physiologic functions. Healthy aging seems associated with modest slowing of gastric emptying of both solids and liquids (**Fig. 5**), but the rate of emptying generally remains within the normal range for young subjects (ie, 1–4 kcal/min).[9,32–36]

There is little information about the effects of aging on the motor activity of the stomach, but fasting antral and duodenal motility does not differ substantially between young and older individuals.[30,37] Although both antegrade and retrograde transpyloric flow pulses are evident after ingestion of a glucose drink in both healthy older and young people, the antegrade flow pulses are less in the older individuals.[9]

Healthy aging is accompanied by loss of enteric neurons and interstitial cells of Cajal throughout the gut; motor function is generally well preserved whereas deficits in sensory function are more apparent. Perception of gastric distension is diminished in the healthy elderly,[31] indicating a reduction in visceral sensitivity. In rodent models of aging, a substantial reduction in the number of neurons in the enteric nervous system is evident (eg, 40% loss in the small intestine in the myenteric plexus of rats).[00] Losses seem selective for cholinergic neurons and involve both the myenteric plexus and the submucous plexus. Nitrergic neurons, which generally mediate inhibitory motor responses, are protected in number but develop axonal swelling, and glial cells are also lost in parallel with neurons.[39] In relation to the extrinsic nerve supply to the gut, the number of vagal fibers innervating the upper gastrointestinal tract does not seem to decline in aging rats, but afferent and efferent fibers undergo morphologic changes. In particular, vagal afferents associated with both the muscle wall and the mucosa of the gut degenerate with age, potentially compromising both sensory feedback and gut reflexes.[40]

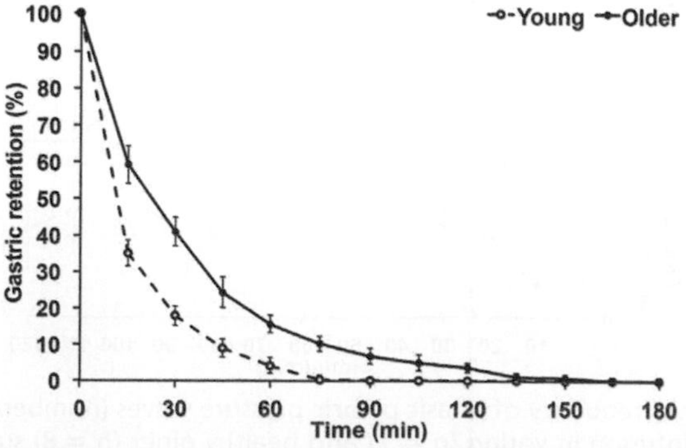

Fig. 5. Mean (±SEM) gastric retention (%) of water consumption (450 mL) in young (n = 8) and healthy older (n = 7) subjects. Gastric emptying of the water was slower in older than in young men, with a mean gastric emptying half-time (T50) of 12 ± 1 minutes in young compared with 23 ± 3 minutes in older adults (*P*<.05).

The good preservation of gastrointestinal motility in the healthy elderly may imply that the large number of neurons in the enteric nervous system provides a considerable functional reserve, but even this may be limited; transit of a radiolabeled meal through the upper gut occurs at a comparable rate in the healthy elderly and the young but is slower through the colon in the elderly, where the loss of enteric neurons is greatest.[41] It may, therefore, not be surprising that constipation is the one gastrointestinal complaint that stands out in the elderly compared with the middle aged.[42]

In addition to mechanical stimuli, perception of chemical stimuli, such as acid, and humoral responses to duodenal nutrient exposure decrease with age. There is evidence for altered responses to the presence of nutrients in the small intestine in older compared with young people, including greater stimulation of phasic pyloric pressure waves by intraduodenal lipid infusion (**Fig. 6**),[43] a greater satiating effect of intraduodenal glucose infusion,[44] and higher fasting and postprandial CCK and GLP-1 concentrations that may contribute to slowing of gastric emptying.[45–49] It is uncertain whether these changes are due to aging and/or reflect changes in nutrient intake. Healthy older people seem to retain their sensitivity to the satiating effects of exogenous GLP-1[48] and may have increased sensitivity to the satiating effects of CCK.[47] Aging is associated with increased postprandial circulating insulin concentrations,[50] mainly due to insulin resistance and associated impaired glucose tolerance,[51] which may reflect increased adiposity and changes in the secretion of incretins, GLP-1 and GIP.[52] There is evidence that the higher prevalence of *Helicobacter pylori* infection and atrophic gastritis in the elderly compared with the young is associated with a decline in levels of the orexigenic peptide ghrelin.[46,53] Plasma concentrations of the anorectic hormone leptin may increase with aging. In women, this may be largely attributable to the increased fat mass that also accompanies aging[54] and in men, the age-related decrease in circulating testosterone concentrations, which is potentiated by obesity.[55]

MEDICAL CONDITIONS AND MEDICATIONS ASSOCIATED WITH DELAYED GASTRIC EMPTYING

Although the effects of healthy aging on gastrointestinal motility are modest, there are numerous comorbidities that increase in prevalence with advancing age and have an impact on gut function, including gastric emptying; Parkinson disease and diabetes

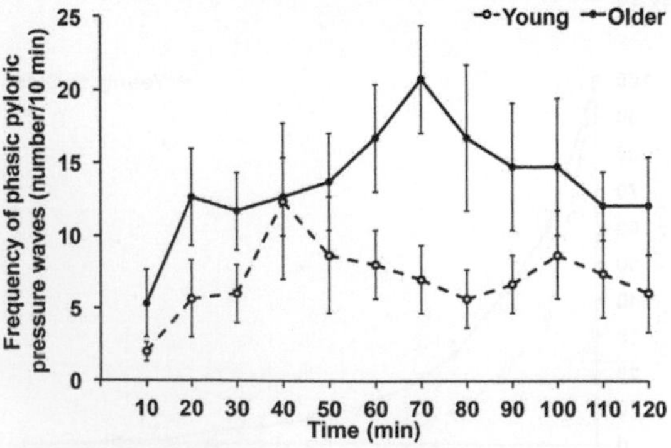

Fig. 6. Mean (±SEM) frequency of phasic pyloric pressure waves (number/10 min) during intraduodenal lipid infusion in young (n = 7) and healthy older (n = 8) subjects. The overall frequency of phasic pyloric pressure waves was greater in the older than young subjects (*P*<.05). (*From* Cook CG, Andrews JM, Jones KL, et al. Effects of small intestinal nutrient infusion on appetite and pyloric motility are modified by age. Am J Physiol 1997;273(2 Pt 2):R758; with permission.)

are typical examples. The relationship of upper gastrointestinal symptoms with the rate of gastric emptying is, however, weak. Administration of several drugs and medical conditions that occur frequently in older people and are associated with acute or chronic delayed gastric emptying are summarized in **Box 2**.

State of nutrition may also affect rate of gastric emptying—concentrations of CCK were higher in undernourished than in well-nourished older subjects,[49] which may potentially result from being undernourished and/or contribute to the undernourished state, and in very young patients with protein energy malnutrition, the gastric emptying half-time of both liquid and semisolid meals was markedly prolonged.[56]

Gastrointestinal dysfunction occurs frequently in Parkinson disease and it is now recognized that abnormalities of gastrointestinal motor function (especially constipation) precede the typical features of Parkinson disease.[57] Involvement of the dorsal motor nucleus of the vagus may influence parasympathetic innervation, whereas abnormalities of the enteric nervous system itself (eg, Lewy bodies and loss of dopaminergic neurons) are also evident. Gastric emptying has been reported to be frequently delayed, even in the absence of levodopa therapy, which in turn slows gastric emptying further. The magnitude of the delay of gastric emptying has been associated with the severity of motor symptoms[58] but not the duration of disease.[59]

IMPLICATIONS FOR THE ABSORPTION OF MEDICATIONS, ENERGY INTAKE, GLYCEMIC CONTROL, AND BLOOD PRESSURE

Delayed gastric emptying may contribute to symptoms, such as nausea and bloating, and result in impaired nutrition and absorption of oral medications.

Box 2
Causes of delayed gastric emptying

Acute

- Critical illness
- Drugs (anticholinergics, calcium channel antagonists, clonidine [an α_2-agonist), levodopa, nitrates, opiates, phosphodiesterase type 5 inhibitors [eg, sildenafil], sumatriptan [a 5HT-1P agonist], tricyclic antidepressants)
- Metabolic (hyperglycemia, hypokalemia)
- Postoperative ileus
- Viral gastroenteritis

Chronic

- Chronic liver disease
- Endocrine and metabolic (diabetes mellitus, hypothyroidism, chronic renal failure, anorexia nervosa)
- Gastroesophageal reflux disease
- HIV infection
- Idiopathic/functional dyspepsia
- Muscular and connective tissue diseases (myotonic dystrophy, muscular dystrophy, dermatomyositis, systemic sclerosis, amyloidosis, tumor associated)
- Postsurgical (including fundoplication)
- Neurologic (central nervous system disease, spinal cord injury, chronic idiopathic intestinal pseudo-obstruction, idiopathic autonomic degeneration)

Slow gastric emptying and alterations in gastric pH (eg, pH higher postprandially in older vs young individuals) may influence the absorption of orally administered medications. For example, a slight reduction in the rate of paracetamol absorption has been reported in healthy older compared with young people.[60] Absorption of benzodiazepines, tetracycline, or levodopa is not, however, significantly altered with age. Also the absorption of nutrients, such as calcium and iron, is reduced with increasing age.[61]

The slowing of gastric emptying with aging may have implications for appetite regulation, potentially contributing to the anorexia of aging. The latter, which may be defined as a reduction of appetite and energy intake in older compared with young adults, predisposes older people to weight loss, particularly loss of skeletal muscle.[62,63] Aging is characterized by attenuated regulation of appetite and energy intake,[30,64,65] so that in the fasting state, appetite and energy intake are less in older than in young adults[43–45,47,62,64] and the suppression of energy intake by nutrients is also less in older than young adults.[30,64] Appetite and energy intake are modulated by central and peripheral influences, the latter including interrelated gastric and small intestinal sensory and motor functions—including variations in gastric emptying[45] and gastric distension[19]—triggered by the interaction with ingested nutrients.

The delayed proximal gastric accommodation to a meal observed in the elderly[31] might contribute to early satiation. Furthermore, in healthy elderly, the antrum is more distended after a nutrient drink—this increase in antral width has been shown to correlate with both satiation and satiety in young and older subjects.[45] Although slower gastric emptying prolongs retention of food in the stomach, favoring satiation, it also delays the onset of powerful satiety signals initiated by the interaction of nutrients with the small intestine. Small intestinal feedback may be modulated by previous patterns of nutrient intake, so that gastric emptying is slower after fasting from nutrients for 4 days,[66] whereas emptying of glucose is more rapid after dietary supplementation with glucose for 3 days.[67] It is, therefore, possible that the slower gastric emptying observed in older individuals may reflect increased small intestinal feedback, occurring as a result of hypersensitivity of small intestinal receptors to nutrients, resulting in, for example, altered gut hormone secretion (CCK, GLP-1, PYY, and GIP) and gut motility,[68] rather than intragastric mechanisms.

Determinants of postprandial glycemia include preprandial blood glucose concentrations, meal composition, the rate of gastric emptying, carbohydrate absorption in the small intestine and incretin release, insulin secretion, and hepatic and peripheral glucose disposal.[3] The rate of gastric emptying, in particular the initial rate of emptying, is now recognized as a critical determinant of the change in blood glucose concentration after a meal,[3,69,70] accounting for approximately 35% of the variance in the initial rise in postprandial glucose levels as well as overall glycemia in healthy individuals.[70] Gastric motility itself is modulated by acute changes in blood glucose concentrations—acute hyperglycemia is associated with a reduction in fundic tone and antral contractions as well as stimulation of pyloric contractions and dysregulation of antroduodenal function, which leads to reversible slowing of gastric emptying. In contrast, a substantial acceleration of gastric emptying occurs during insulin-induced hypoglycemia (blood glucose levels approximately 2.6 mmol/L). Moreover, changes in gastric emptying within the physiologic range of blood glucose concentrations have also been noted, such that gastric emptying of both solids and liquids is faster when the blood glucose concentration is 4 mmol/L than when it is 8 mmol/L in healthy individuals.

Disordered motor function involving all segments of the gastrointestinal tract occurs in up to 50% of patients with long-standing types 1 and 2 diabetes mellitus.[3]

Disordered gastric emptying contributes to upper gut symptoms and may result in, and also arise from, poor glycemic control. Although a delay in gastric emptying may improve the postprandial blood glucose profile in non–insulin-requiring patients due to a slower delivery of carbohydrate to the small intestine and is a therapeutic target for short-acting GLP-1 agonists, such as exenatide,[71] it results in a mismatch between the absorption of glucose and the onset of insulin action in patients receiving exogenous insulin.

Blood pressure can decrease markedly after meals in older people—a phenomenon known as postprandial hypotension—and this represents an important, but generally under-recognized, clinical problem.[72]

Postprandial hypotension, defined as a fall in systolic blood pressure of greater than 20 mm Hg, or a decrease to 90 mm Hg when the preprandial systolic blood pressure is greater than or equal to 100 mm Hg, within 2 hours of a meal,[73] is associated with several sequelae that have an adverse impact on quality of life as well as increased mortality. The most common manifestations seem to be syncope, falls, angina, dizziness, nausea, light-headedness, and/or visual disturbance. Hypertensive subjects exhibit greater reductions in postprandial blood pressure compared with age-matched normotensive subjects,[72] and older people with type 2 diabetes mellitus and Parkinson disease are at particular risk. The prevalence of postprandial hypotension is 24% to 38% in healthy community-dwelling elderly and recipients of residential care, 20% to 91% in hospitalized geriatric patients, approximately 40% in type 2 diabetes mellitus patients, and 40% to 100% in Parkinson disease patients.[72]

Recent studies indicate that postprandial hypotension should, in the broadest sense, be regarded as a gastrointestinal disorder, because the magnitude of the postprandial decline in blood pressure depends on the regulation of splanchnic blood flow, gastric distension, and the release of gastrointestinal hormones related to both the rate of gastric emptying and the small intestinal response to ingested nutrients. Postprandial hypotension is less likely to occur with higher-volume, low-calorie meals, and the macronutrient content may influence the timing of the fall in blood pressure. Among the macronutrients, carbohydrate, in particular, contributes to a fall in blood pressure.[74] After oral or small intestinal administration of glucose, the magnitude of the fall in blood pressure is related to the rate at which glucose enters the small intestine.[69] Furthermore, a recent study has demonstrated that healthy subjects with postprandial hypotension have, as a group, more rapid gastric emptying (**Fig. 7**).[75] Dietary

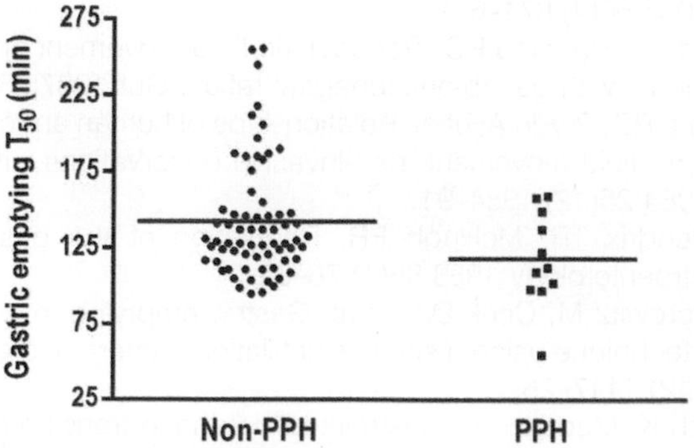

Fig. 7. Gastric emptying half-times (T_{50}) in subjects without (n = 68, ●) and with (n = 11, ■) postprandial hypotension (PPH) (P<.05). (*From* Trahair LG, Horowitz M, Jones KL. Postprandial hypotension is associated with more rapid gastric emptying in healthy older subjects. J Am Med Dir Assoc 2015;[Epub ahead of print]; with permission.)

and pharmacologic approaches to slow gastric emptying and small intestinal carbohydrate absorption (eg, the α-glucosidase inhibitor acarbose or dietary interventions, such as smaller but more frequent meals) may prove effective in the treatment of postprandial hypotension,[76] whereas distending the stomach (eg, by drinking a glass of water[77]), postprandial exercise, and modifying meal temperature may attenuate the fall.[72] Accordingly, the fall in blood pressure induced by oral glucose may be less when intragastric volume is relatively higher as a result of increased gastric distension.

In summary, aging is characterized by modest slowing of gastric emptying, which is relevant to the absorption of oral medications as well as the regulation of appetite, postprandial glycemia, and blood pressure.

REFERENCES

1. Deloose E, Janssen P, Depoortere I, et al. The migrating motor complex: control mechanisms and its role in health and disease. Nat Rev Gastroenterol Hepatol 2012;9(5):271–85.
2. Stevens JE, Jones KL, Rayner CK, et al. Pathophysiology and pharmacotherapy of gastroparesis: current and future perspectives. Expert Opin Pharmacother 2013;14(9):1171–86.
3. Phillips LK, Deane AM, Jones KL, et al. Gastric emptying and glycaemia in health and diabetes mellitus. Nat Rev Endocrinol 2014;11:112–28.
4. Horowitz M, Dent J, Fraser R, et al. Role and integration of mechanisms controlling gastric emptying. Dig Dis Sci 1994;39(12 Suppl):7S–13S.
5. Horowitz M, Dent J. Disordered gastric emptying: mechanical basis, assessment and treatment. Baillieres Clin Gastroenterol 1991;5(2):371–407.
6. Heddle R, Collins PJ, Dent J, et al. Motor mechanisms associated with slowing of the gastric emptying of a solid meal by an intraduodenal lipid infusion. J Gastroenterol Hepatol 1989;4(5):437–47.
7. Meyer JH, Ohashi H, Jehn D, et al. Size of liver particles emptied from the human stomach. Gastroenterology 1981;80(6):1489–96.
8. Rees WD, Go VL, Malagelada JR. Antroduodenal motor response to solid-liquid and homogenized meals. Gastroenterology 1979;76(6):1438–42.
9. O'Donovan D, Hausken T, Lei Y, et al. Effect of aging on transpyloric flow, gastric emptying, and intragastric distribution in healthy humans–impact on glycemia. Dig Dis Sci 2005;50(4):671–6.
10. King PM, Pryde A, Heading RC. Transpyloric fluid movement and antroduodenal motility in patients with gastro-oesophageal reflux. Gut 1987;28(5):545–8.
11. King PM, Adam RD, Pryde A, et al. Relationships of human antroduodenal motility and transpyloric fluid movement: non-invasive observations with real-time ultrasound. Gut 1984;25(12):1384–91.
12. Brener W, Hendrix TR, McHugh PR. Regulation of the gastric emptying of glucose. Gastroenterology 1983;85(1):76–82.
13. Collins PJ, Horowitz M, Cook DJ, et al. Gastric emptying in normal subjects–a reproducible technique using a single scintillation camera and computer system. Gut 1983;24(12):1117–25.
14. Graff J, Brinch K, Madsen JL. Gastrointestinal mean transit times in young and middle-aged healthy subjects. Clin Physiol 2001;21(2):253–9.
15. Teff KL, Alavi A, Chen J, et al. Muscarinic blockade inhibits gastric emptying of mixed-nutrient meal: effects of weight and gender. Am J Physiol 1999;276(3 Pt 2):R707–14.

16. Camilleri M, Malagelada JR, Brown ML, et al. Relation between antral motility and gastric emptying of solids and liquids in humans. Am J Physiol 1985;249(5 Pt 1): G580–5.
17. Malbert CH, Ruckebusch Y. Relationships between pressure and flow across the gastroduodenal junction in dogs. Am J Physiol 1991;260(4 Pt 1):G653–7.
18. Collins PJ, Houghton LA, Read NW, et al. Role of the proximal and distal stomach in mixed solid and liquid meal emptying. Gut 1991;32(6):615–9.
19. Horowitz M, Maddox A, Bochner M, et al. Relationships between gastric emptying of solid and caloric liquid meals and alcohol absorption. Am J Physiol 1989;257(2 Pt 1):G291–8.
20. Goyal RK, Hirano I. The enteric nervous system. N Engl J Med 1996;334(17): 1106–15.
21. Wu T, Rayner CK, Young RL, et al. Gut motility and enteroendocrine secretion. Curr Opin Pharmacol 2013;13(6):928–34.
22. Jones KL, Doran SM, Hveem K, et al. Relation between postprandial satiation and antral area in normal subjects. Am J Clin Nutr 1997;66(1):127–32.
23. Ohno T, Mochiki E, Kuwano H. The roles of motilin and ghrelin in gastrointestinal motility. Int J Peptides 2010;2010 [pii: 820794].
24. Camilleri M, Shin A. Novel and validated approaches for gastric emptying scintigraphy in patients with suspected gastroparesis. Dig Dis Sci 2013;58(7):1813–5.
25. Parkman HP, Hasler WL, Fisher RS. American Gastroenterological Association technical review on the diagnosis and treatment of gastroparesis. Gastroenterology 2004;127(5):1592–622.
26. Phillips LK, Rayner CK, Jones KL, et al. Measurement of gastric emptying in diabetes. J Diabet Complications 2014;28(6):894–903.
27. Bolondi L, Bortolotti M, Santi V, et al. Measurement of gastric emptying time by real-time ultrasonography. Gastroenterology 1985;89(4):752–9.
28. Gilja OH, Hausken T, degaard S, et al. Gastric emptying measured by ultrasonography. World J Gastroenterol 1999;5(2):93–4.
29. Gilja OH, Detmer PR, Jong JM, et al. Intragastric distribution and gastric emptying assessed by three-dimensional ultrasonography. Gastroenterology 1997;113(1):38–49.
30. Soenen S, Giezenaar C, Hutchison AT, et al. Effects of intraduodenal protein on appetite, energy intake, and antropyloroduodenal motility in healthy older compared with young men in a randomized trial. Am J Clin Nutr 2014;100(4):1108–15.
31. Rayner CK, MacIntosh CG, Chapman IM, et al. Effects of age on proximal gastric motor and sensory function. Scand J Gastroenterol 2000;35(10):1041–7.
32. Clarkston WK, Pantano MM, Morley JE, et al. Evidence for the anorexia of aging: gastrointestinal transit and hunger in healthy elderly vs. young adults. Am J Physiol Regul Integr Comp Physiol 1997;272(1):R243–8.
33. Wegener M, Borsch G, Schaffstein J, et al. Effect of ageing on the gastrointestinal transit of a lactulose-supplemented mixed solid-liquid meal in humans. Digestion 1988;39(1):40–6.
34. Horowitz M, Maddern GJ, Chatterton BE, et al. Changes in gastric emptying rates with age. Clin Sci (Lond) 1984;67(2):213–8.
35. Moore JG, Tweedy C, Christian PE, et al. Effect of age on gastric emptying of liquid–solid meals in man. Dig Dis Sci 1983;28(4):340–4.
36. Evans MA, Triggs EJ, Cheung M, et al. Gastric emptying rate in the elderly: implications for drug therapy. J Am Geriatr Soc 1981;29(5):201–5.
37. Fich A, Camilleri M, Phillips SF. Effect of age on human gastric and small bowel motility. J Clin Gastroenterol 1989;11(4):416–20.

38. Wade PR. Aging and neural control of the GI tract. I. Age-related changes in the enteric nervous system. Am J Physiol Gastrointest Liver Physiol 2002;283(3): G489–95.
39. Phillips RJ, Powley TL. Innervation of the gastrointestinal tract: patterns of aging. Auton Neurosci 2007;136(1–2):1–19.
40. Phillips RJ, Walter GC, Powley TL. Age-related changes in vagal afferents innervating the gastrointestinal tract. Auton Neurosci 2010;153(1–2):90–8.
41. Madsen JL, Graff J. Effects of ageing on gastrointestinal motor function. Age Ageing 2004;33(2):154–9.
42. Camilleri M, Cowen T, Koch TR. Enteric neurodegeneration in ageing. Neurogastroenterol Motil 2008;20(3):185–96.
43. Cook CG, Andrews JM, Jones KL, et al. Effects of small intestinal nutrient infusion on appetite and pyloric motility are modified by age. Am J Physiol 1997; 273(2 Pt 2):R755–61.
44. MacIntosh CG, Horowitz M, Verhagen MA, et al. Effect of small intestinal nutrient infusion on appetite, gastrointestinal hormone release, and gastric myoelectrical activity in young and older men. Am J Gastroenterol 2001;96(4):997–1007.
45. Sturm K, Parker B, Wishart J, et al. Energy intake and appetite are related to antral area in healthy young and older subjects. Am J Clin Nutr 2004;80(3): 656–67.
46. Sturm K, MacIntosh CG, Parker BA, et al. Appetite, food intake, and plasma concentrations of cholecystokinin, ghrelin, and other gastrointestinal hormones in undernourished older women and well-nourished young and older women. J Clin Endocrinol Metab 2003;88(8):3747–55.
47. MacIntosh CG, Morley JE, Wishart J, et al. Effect of exogenous cholecystokinin (CCK)-8 on food intake and plasma CCK, leptin, and insulin concentrations in older and young adults: evidence for increased CCK activity as a cause of the anorexia of aging. J Clin Endocrinol Metab 2001;86(12):5830–7.
48. Gutzwiller JP, Goke B, Drewe J, et al. Glucagon-like peptide-1: a potent regulator of food intake in humans. Gut 1999;44(1):81–6.
49. Berthelemy P, Bouisson M, Vellas B, et al. Postprandial cholecystokinin secretion in elderly with protein-energy undernutrition. J Am Geriatr Soc 1992;40(4):365–9.
50. Fraze E, Chiou YA, Chen YD, et al. Age-related changes in postprandial plasma glucose, insulin, and free fatty acid concentrations in nondiabetic individuals. J Am Geriatr Soc 1987;35(3):224–8.
51. Scheen AJ. Diabetes mellitus in the elderly: insulin resistance and/or impaired insulin secretion? Diabetes Metab 2005;31(Spec No 2). P. 5S27–5S34.
52. Trahair LG, Horowitz M, Rayner CK, et al. Comparative effects of variations in duodenal glucose load on glycemic, insulinemic, and incretin responses in healthy young and older subjects. J Clin Endocrinol Metab 2012;97(3):844–51.
53. Salles N. Basic mechanisms of the aging gastrointestinal tract. Dig Dis 2007; 25(2):112–7.
54. Baumgartner RN, Waters DL, Morley JE, et al. Age-related changes in sex hormones affect the sex difference in serum leptin independently of changes in body fat. Metabolism 1999;48(3):378–84.
55. Hislop MS, Ratanjee BD, Soule SG, et al. Effects of anabolic-androgenic steroid use or gonadal testosterone suppression on serum leptin concentration in men. Eur J Endocrinol 1999;141(1):40–6.
56. Shaaban SY, Nassar MF, Sawaby AS, et al. Ultrasonographic gastric emptying in protein energy malnutrition: effect of type of meal and nutritional recovery. Eur J Clin Nutr 2004;58(6):972–8.

57. Pfeiffer RF. Gastrointestinal dysfunction in Parkinson's disease. Lancet Neurol 2003;2(2):107–16.
58. Goetze O, Nikodem AB, Wiezcorek J, et al. Predictors of gastric emptying in Parkinson's disease. Neurogastroenterol Motil 2006;18(5):369–75.
59. Tanaka Y, Kato T, Nishida H, et al. Is there a delayed gastric emptying of patients with early-stage, untreated Parkinson's disease? An analysis using the 13C-acetate breath test. J Neurol 2011;258(3):421–6.
60. Divoll M, Ameer B, Abernethy DR, et al. Age does not alter acetaminophen absorption. J Am Geriatr Soc 1982;30(4):240–4.
61. Bender AD. Effect of age on intestinal absorption: implications for drug absorption in the elderly. J Am Geriatr Soc 1968;16(12):1331–9.
62. Soenen S, Chapman IM. Body weight, anorexia, and undernutrition in older people. J Am Med Dir Assoc 2013;14:642–8.
63. Morley JE, Silver AJ. Anorexia in the elderly. Neurobiol Aging 1988;9(1):9–16.
64. Rolls BJ, Dimeo KA, Shide DJ. Age-related impairments in the regulation of food intake. Am J Clin Nutr 1995;62(5):923–31.
65. Roberts SB, Fuss P, Heyman MB, et al. Control of food intake in older men. JAMA 1994;272(20):1601–6.
66. Corvilain B, Abramowicz M, Fery F, et al. Effect of short-term starvation on gastric emptying in humans: relationship to oral glucose tolerance. Am J Physiol 1995; 269(4 Pt 1):G512–7.
67. Cunningham KM, Horowitz M, Read NW. The effect of short-term dietary supplementation with glucose on gastric emptying in humans. Br J Nutr 1991;65(1): 15–9.
68. Seimon RV, Lange K, Little TJ, et al. Pooled-data analysis identifies pyloric pressures and plasma cholecystokinin concentrations as major determinants of acute energy intake in healthy, lean men. Am J Clin Nutr 2010;92(1):61–8.
69. O'Donovan D, Feinle C, Tonkin A, et al. Postprandial hypotension in response to duodenal glucose delivery in healthy older subjects. J Physiol 2002;540(Pt 2): 673–9.
70. Horowitz M, Edelbroek MA, Wishart JM, et al. Relationship between oral glucose tolerance and gastric emptying in normal healthy subjects. Diabetologia 1993; 36(9):857–62.
71. Linnebjerg H, Park S, Kothare PA, et al. Effect of exenatide on gastric emptying and relationship to postprandial glycemia in type 2 diabetes. Regul Pept 2008; 151(1–3):123–9.
72. Trahair LG, Horowitz M, Jones KL. Postprandial hypotension: a systematic review. J Am Med Dir Assoc 2014;15(6):394–409.
73. Jansen RW, Lipsitz LA. Postprandial hypotension: epidemiology, pathophysiology, and clinical management. Ann Intern Med 1995;122(4):286–95.
74. Visvanathan R, Horowitz M, Chapman I. The hypotensive response to oral fat is comparable but slower compared with carbohydrate in healthy elderly subjects. Br J Nutr 2006;95(2):340–5.
75. Trahair LG, Horowitz M, Jones KL. Postprandial hypotension is associated with more rapid gastric emptying in healthy older subjects. J Am Med Dir Assoc 2015. [Epub ahead of print].
76. Gentilcore D, Bryant B, Wishart JM, et al. Acarbose attenuates the hypotensive response to sucrose and slows gastric emptying in the elderly. Am J Med 2005;118(11):1289.
77. Shannon JR, Diedrich A, Biaggioni I, et al. Water drinking as a treatment for orthostatic syndromes. Am J Med 2002;112(5):355–60.

Vitamin Supplementation in the Elderly

Seema Joshi, MD[a,b,*]

KEYWORDS

- Aged • Antioxidants • Dietary supplements • Health status
- Vitamins/administration and dosage • Nutritional requirements

KEY POINTS

- Older individuals, especially those with associated risk factors, may be at a high risk for developing certain vitamin deficiencies.
- Presentation of vitamin-related disorders may be atypical or masked by coexisting diseases or a failure to thrive.
- Use of vitamin supplements is very common in the elderly, making them vulnerable to drug--nutrient interactions.
- Current clinical trials on vitamin supplements for promotion of health and prevention of disease have failed to demonstrate the strong associations seen in observational studies.

VITAMINS AND AGING

Activity levels and energy requirements decrease with aging. Consequently, there is a reduction in total energy intake along with a decline in nutrient intake, including vitamins and minerals.[1,2] Vitamin requirements continue to change over the life span. There is strong evidence of an increase in the requirements for vitamins D, B6, and B12 in the elderly. B12 levels decline significantly with aging, in large part due to a high prevalence of atrophic gastritis. Vitamin D requirements increase with age as well. This increase seems to result from a diminished cutaneous synthesis of vitamin D by aging skin and decreased sun exposure, particularly in the elderly in institutionalized settings.[3,4]

This material is the result of work supported with resources and the use of facilities at the Dwight D. Eisenhower Veterans Affairs Medical Center, Leavenworth, KS, USA.
[a] Department of Geriatrics and Extended Care, Dwight D. Eisenhower Veterans Affairs Medical Center, 4101 South 4th Street Traffic way, Leavenworth, KS 66048, USA; [b] Division of Health Services Research, Department of Internal Medicine, University of Kansas Medical Center, 4043 Wescoe, MS 1037, 3901 Rainbow Boulevard, Kansas City, KS 66160, USA
* Dwight D. Eisenhower VAMC, B-122, R323C, 4101 South 4th Street Traffic way, Leavenworth, KS 66048.
E-mail address: seema.joshi@va.gov

Clin Geriatr Med 31 (2015) 355–366
http://dx.doi.org/10.1016/j.cger.2015.04.004
0749-0690/15/$ – see front matter Published by Elsevier Inc.

Multiple factors have been implicated in the development of undernutrition in the elderly. Polypharmacy is common, and long-term administration of some medications may adversely affect vitamin status. Also, in this population, presentation of vitamin disorders is usually atypical or masked by coexisting diseases or a failure to thrive.[5,6]

Table 1 summarizes the risk factors contributing to micronutrient deficiencies, and **Table 2** lists medications that adversely affect the vitamin levels.

There has been an increased interest in the use of vitamins for health and disease prevention. Almost 20% to 60% of the elderly consume vitamin supplements, increasing the potential for toxicity and likelihood of drug-nutrient interactions.[7]

VITAMIN SUPPLEMENTATION AND DISEASE PREVENTION

Vitamins are organic compounds required in the diet in small amounts for the maintenance of normal metabolic integrity. However, vitamin D and niacin do not comply with this definition of vitamins. Vitamin D is synthesized in the skin from 7-dehydrocholesterol on exposure to sunlight, and niacin can be formed from the essential amino acid, tryptophan.

Vitamins have been categorized as fat soluble or water soluble. Vitamins A, D, E, and K are fat soluble and the remaining (vitamins B1, B2, B6, B12, niacin, biotin, and vitamin C) are water soluble. Vitamins A, C, E, and β-carotene are also referred to as antioxidant vitamins and have been suggested to limit oxidative damage in humans.[7,8]

VITAMIN A AND β-CAROTENE

Vitamin A consists of preformed vitamin A (retinol) and the carotenoids such as β-carotene. Vitamin A refers to preformed retinol and the carotenoids that are converted to retinol.

Table 1
Risk factors for altered vitamin status in the elderly

Medical factors	• Medications: Proton pump inhibitors, H2 antagonists, cholestyramine, INH (Isoniazid), metformin, sulfasalazine, rifampin, anticonvulsants, and colchicine • Disorders of absorption: Atrophic gastritis, bacterial overgrowth of bowel, terminal ileal resection, gluten enteropathy, lactose intolerance • Dysphagia: Neurologic disorders, esophageal strictures/webs, esophagitis, malignancy, achalasia, scleroderma • Malignancies • Neurologic disorders affecting intake: Dementia and related disorders, strokes, tremors • Altered dentition
Psychological factors	• Depression • Alcoholism • Late life paranoia • Dementia
Social factors	• Social isolation • Impaired IADLs (Instrumental Activities of Daily Living) • Financial problems
Physiologic factors	• Sensory impairment: Altered vision, olfaction, taste • Anorexia of aging

Adapted from Joshi S, Morley JE. Vitamins and minerals. Principles and practice of geriatric medicine. 5th edition. UK: John Wiley & Sons; 2012. p. 220; with permission.

Table 2
Medications affecting vitamin status

Medication	Vitamins	Mechanisms of Interaction
Anticonvulsants: Phenytoin, phenobarbital, primidone	Vitamin D	Induction of CYP enzyme 3A4 with resultant metabolism of vitamin D to inactive compounds.
Metformin	Vitamin B12	Poor absorption in the ileum due to competition with the calcium-dependent intrinsic factor
Proton pump inhibitors	Vitamin B12	Decreased gastric acid resulting in decreased cleavage of protein-bound B12 and absorption
Cholestyramine	Vitamin D, E, and folate	Decreases absorption by adsorption of nutrient
Colchicine	Vitamin B12	Inhibits development of vitamin B12 receptor in the ileum
Rifampin	Vitamin D	Induction of hepatic enzymes and metabolism of vitamin D to inactive metabolites
Sulfasalazine	Folate	Inhibits folate absorption by interfering with the breakdown of dietary folate
Isoniazid	Pyridoxine (vitamin B6)	Competes with vitamin B6 in its action as a cofactor in the synthesis of synaptic neurotransmitters
Corticosteroids	Vitamin D	Inhibit vitamin D-mediated actions on calcium
Levodopa	All vitamins	Induce anorexia and poor intake
Methotrexate	Folate	Binds to and inhibits dihydrofolate reductase, inhibiting the formation of reduced folates
Alcohol	Vitamin B1, B2, B6, and folate	Insufficient intake, reduced gastrointestinal absorption, or reduced storage. Also, increased breakdown of pyridoxine during ethanol metabolism and urinary excretion of folate

Adapted from Hamrick I, Counts SH. Vitamin and mineral supplements. Prim Care Clin Office Prac 2008;35:729–47; with permission.

Natural sources include yellow, orange, and red plant compounds, such as carrots and green leafy vegetables. Preformed vitamin A is found only in animal products, including organ meats, fish, egg yolks, and fortified milk.

Vitamin A intake decreases with age; however, deficiency is uncommon even in the very old, and underlying chronic renal impairment increases the risk of toxicity with supplementation.[9]

Cancer Prevention

The results from observational and randomized clinical trials on cancer prevention have been inconsistent. The benefits seen in observational studies of dietary vitamin A most likely represent the effects of β-carotene. Randomized, double-blind, placebo-controlled trials, such as the Alpha-Tocopherol, Beta Carotene Cancer (ATBC) Prevention Study and Beta Carotene and Retinol Efficacy Trial (CARET), have shown an increased risk of lung cancer among men receiving the supplements. The Physicians' Health Study did not demonstrate an effect of β-carotene supplementation on lung cancer or overall mortality among 22,071 men aged 40 to 84 years after an average follow-up of 12 years.[10,11]

There was a modest but statistically nonsignificant increase in risk of prostate cancer among β-carotene recipients in the ATBC Study; this was reduced in the early posttrial period and absent in the later posttrial years. Also, there was no effect of β-carotene in the CARET and Physicians' Health Study on the risk of prostate cancer.[12,13]

There are no clinical trials on vitamin A intake and risk of breast cancer, and results of observational studies have not been consistent. Data from the Nurses' Health Study have suggested that a high intake of carotenoids may decrease the risk of breast cancer, particularly in women with a positive family history.[14,15]

The Polyp Prevention Study Group did not show any efficacy of supplemental β-carotene and vitamins C and E in the prevention of colorectal cancer.[16]

Cataracts/Macular Degeneration

The Physician Health Study found no effect of vitamin A supplements on the overall risk of cataract formation; it did reduce the risk significantly among smokers though.[17] The Age-Related Eye Disease Study demonstrated that daily oral supplementation with antioxidant vitamins and minerals reduced the risk of developing advanced age-related macular degeneration (AMD) by 25% at 5 years.[18] However, subsequent meta-analyses have found no preventive effects of antioxidant supplements in general, or of β-carotene or α-tocopherol specifically, to prevent or delay the onset of AMD.[19–21]

Bone Health

The incidence of osteoporotic fractures has been found to be unusually high in areas where dietary intake of vitamin A (retinol) is high. Vitamin A intake seems to be associated with reduced bone mineral density and osteoporosis. Current evidence from observational studies consistently suggests that vitamin A intakes greater than 1500 μg/d are a risk factor for osteopenia and fractures.[22,23]

VITAMIN E

Vitamin E occurs in 8 natural forms as tocopherols (α, β, γ, and δ) and tocotrienols (α, β, γ, and δ), all of which possess potent antioxidant properties.

Primary sources of vitamin E are vegetable oil, wheat germ, leafy vegetables, egg yolk, margarine, and legumes.

Deficiency of vitamin E is uncommon in humans except in unusual circumstances such as fat malabsorption.

Vitamin E deficiency can be measured by examining serum or tissue α-tocopherol levels.[24,25]

Cancer Prevention

The protective effect of vitamin E seen in observational studies has not been supported by randomized trials. The decreased incidence of prostate cancer and associated mortality seen in the ATBC study has not been demonstrated in subsequent trials. The SELECT trial, the Physicians' Health Study II, Heart Outcomes Prevention Evaluation (HOPE) -TOO trial, and the Women's Antioxidant Cardiovascular Study found no effect of vitamin E supplementation on cancer incidence or cancer deaths.[18,26–28]

Cardiovascular Disease

Vitamin E supplementation was thought to be protective against cardiovascular disease as suggested by the Nurses' Health Study and another large study on men.[29,30] Subsequent clinical trials have not shown any benefit in either primary or secondary prevention of Coronary Heart Disease. The ATBC study did not show any effect of vitamin E supplementation on stroke risk. A subsequent subgroup analysis suggested the possibility of an increased risk of subarachnoid hemorrhage and a decreased risk for ischemic stroke. The HOPE trial did not show any effect of vitamin E on progression of carotid intimal medial thickness, and the HOPE-TOO trial showed an increase in heart failure.[31–33]

Dementia

Data from observational studies have suggested that increased dietary intake of vitamin E may have a protective effect against the development of Alzheimer disease and vascular dementia.[34,35] A randomized trial of selegiline, vitamin E, both, or placebo among patients with Alzheimer disease showed that both selegiline and vitamin E were independently associated with significant reductions in several outcomes, including functional decline.[36] However, subsequent randomized trials of vitamin E supplementation in patients with mild cognitive impairment or in healthy older women have not shown any cognitive benefits.[37,38]

All-Cause Mortality

A meta-analysis of 19 randomized clinical trials examining the dose-response relationship between vitamin E and overall mortality found that vitamin E supplementation with a dose of 400 IU or more per day was associated with a significantly increased risk of all-cause mortality.[39]

VITAMIN C

Vitamin C (ascorbic acid) is a water-soluble vitamin widely found in citrus fruits, raw leafy vegetables, strawberries, melons, tomatoes, broccoli, and peppers.

Vitamin C deficiency is common in many frail elderly populations. Manifestations of deficiency may be attributed to age-related physiologic changes in the elderly.[40,41]

High doses of vitamin C have been associated with fatal cardiac arrhythmias in patients with iron overload.[42]

Studies evaluating the effects of vitamin C in cancer and cardiovascular disease have shown no beneficial effects.[43,44]

Cataracts

Data on the effect of vitamin C on cataracts have been conflicting. The Nurses' Health Study showed a 45% reduction in the risk of cataracts requiring extraction in women using vitamin C supplements for at least 10 years. However, a randomized, placebo-controlled study of supplementation with high-dose vitamins C and E and β-carotene found no reduction in the 7-year risk of development or progression of age-related lens opacities with vitamin C supplementation.[45,46]

Common Cold

Regular supplementation trials have shown that vitamin C reduces the duration of colds. However, a meta-analysis of 29 trials involving 11,306 participants taking vitamin C supplements on a regular basis did not show a reduction in the incidence of colds in the general population. Nevertheless, the study did reveal a 50% decrease in the incidence of cold in patients exposed to vigorous activity, especially in extreme conditions.[47]

VITAMIN D

Vitamin D, or calciferol, refers to a group of lipid-soluble compounds with a 4-ringed cholesterol backbone.

It is not a true vitamin because humans are able to synthesize it with adequate sunlight exposure.

It is derived primarily via synthesis in the skin. Dietary sources include fortified milk, milk products, oily fish, egg yolks, and fortified foods.

Calcidiol levels are used to assess vitamin D status.[41]

Osteoporosis

The benefits of calcium and vitamin D supplements on bone mineral density and reduction in risk of all fracture types have been demonstrated in multiple randomized controlled trials. The DIPART (vitamin D Individual Patient Analysis of Randomized Trials) group has since revealed that both calcium and vitamin D supplementation together, and not vitamin D alone, reduced hip and total fractures.[48–50]

Falls

Several studies have examined the dose-response relationship between falls and vitamin D supplementation. A meta-analysis of double-blinded, randomized, controlled trials of older individuals, looking specifically at supplemental vitamin D in the prevention of falls, found that supplemental vitamin D in a dose of 700 to 1000 IU a day reduced the risk of falling among older individuals by 19%. It also concluded that vitamin D doses of less than 700 IU or serum 25-hydroxyvitamin D (25[OH]D) concentrations lower than 60 nmol/L may not reduce the risk of falls among older individuals.[51]

However, 2 separate studies that used annual high-dose vitamin D supplements in elderly men and women showed an increased risk of falls and fracture. These studies point to the need to evaluate safe dose regimens for vitamin D.[52,53]

Cardiovascular Disease

A meta-analysis of 19 prospective studies revealed an inverse relationship between serum 25(OH)D levels (ranging from 8 to 24 ng/mL) and risk of cardiovascular disease (relative risk of 1.03, 95% confidence interval 1.00–1.60, per 10 ng/mL decrement in serum 25[OH]D).[54] However, there was no effect of supplementation on cardiovascular outcomes, including myocardial infarction and stroke in intervention trials.[55] Observational data show that, in normotensive and hypertensive individuals, there is an inverse association between 25(OH)D concentration and blood pressure.[56] A meta-analysis of 8 randomized trials examining the effects of vitamin D supplementation on blood pressure in hypertensive men and women showed a small but significant reduction in diastolic blood pressure and a nonsignificant reduction in systolic blood pressure.[57]

Cancer

Observational studies have suggested a link between poor vitamin D status and risk of nearly all cancers. A reanalysis by a World Health Organization working group identified the highest risk of colon cancer associated with a poor vitamin D status.[58,59] Despite these observations, results of vitamin D intervention trials on cancer risk have been inconsistent. In the Women's Health Initiative, treatment with vitamin D3 and calcium did not have an effect on the incidence of colorectal cancer.[60] A recent meta-analysis of 18 randomized trials did not reveal any effect of vitamin D supplementation on the incidence of cancer among older community-dwelling women. Vitamin D3 supplementation seemed to decrease cancer mortality, and vitamin D supplementation decreased all-cause mortality.[61]

Diabetes

Observational studies show an inverse relationship between circulating 25(OH)D levels and the risk of diabetes. However, intervention studies either have been negative or have shown only limited beneficial effects.[62,63]

FOLIC ACID

Folates represent a group of related pterin compounds. More than 35 forms of the vitamin are found naturally.

The various dietary sources include green leafy vegetables, fresh fruits, yeast, and liver and other organ meats.

Folate deficiency can be determined on the basis of decreased serum folate levels; however, red cell folate level may be a better indicator if there has been a recent dietary change.

Cancer

Observational studies suggest that sufficient folate intake might prevent cancers in certain at risk populations. Benefits have not been confirmed in clinical trials and have raised the possibility of harm.[64–66]

Cardiovascular Disease

Elevated homocysteine levels are associated with an increased risk of cardiovascular disease, and supplementation with folic acid can lower homocysteine levels. However, benefits of supplementation with folic acid for secondary prevention of cardiovascular disease have not been seen in meta-analysis of randomized trials.[67,68]

VITAMIN B2

Riboflavin, or vitamin B2, is an important component of the coenzymes flavin mononucleotide and Flavin adenine dinucleotide.

Dietary sources include dairy products, green leafy vegetables, whole and enriched grains, meats, liver, poultry, and fish. It is not destroyed by heat, oxidation, or acid but is susceptible to ultraviolet light and alkalis.

Vitamin B2 deficiency is regarded as the most common vitamin deficiency in the United States. There is some evidence that the requirements for riboflavin may increase with aging.

Erythrocyte glutathione reductase assay is a better test for riboflavin deficiency because plasma concentrations tend to reflect recent dietary intake.[48,69]

Vitamin B2 supplementation helps only in the prevention of deficiency.

VITAMIN B6

Vitamin B6 comprises various derivatives of pyridine, including pyridoxine, pyridoxal, and pyridoxamine.

Dietary sources include meats, whole grains, vegetables, and nuts.

Dietary deficiency is rare; however, there is evidence that the requirements are increased in the elderly.

Long-term use with doses exceeding 200 mg per day (in adults) may cause peripheral neuropathies and photosensitivity.

Observational evidence reveals a lower risk of colorectal and breast cancer associated with higher plasma levels of vitamin B6. There is currently no evidence supporting the role of vitamin B6 supplementation in cancer prevention.[70,71]

VITAMIN B12

Vitamin B12 is a group of cobalamin compounds that have a corrin ring with a cobalt atom at the center.

A deficiency of cobalamin leads to an increase in homocysteine and methyl-malonic acid.

Vitamin B12 deficiency may be seen in the elderly population as documented by elevated methyl-malonic acid with or without elevated total homocysteine concentrations in combination with low or low-normal vitamin B12 concentrations.

Low vitamin B12 serum levels are associated with poor cognitive function, cognitive decline, and dementia. However, randomized controlled trials do not provide any clear evidence that supplementation with vitamin B12 improves dementia or slows cognitive decline.[72]

Elevated homocysteine levels are associated with an increased risk of cardiovascular disease. However, lowering homocysteine levels with folate and vitamin B6 and B12 supplementation has not been shown to prevent cardiovascular disease.

SUMMARY

Epidemiologic associations of vitamin supplements in health promotion and disease prevention have not been supported by clinical trials. However, a diet rich in vitamins seems to be associated with improved health. Aging is associated with a reduced caloric intake, thus increasing the risk of micronutrient deficiencies. At the same time, the elderly are also at risk of toxicity from excessive doses of vitamin supplements and are vulnerable to drug nutrient interactions. Both toxicity and deficiency may have atypical presentations and may be masked by underlying coexisting conditions. Use of vitamin D supplements in elderly at risk for falls and vitamin supplements among those at risk for micronutrient deficiencies may be recommended. However, current evidence does not support the use of vitamin supplements to promote health or prevent aging.

REFERENCES

1. Briefel RR, Johnson CL. Secular trends in dietary intake in the United States. Annu Rev Nutr 2004;24:401–31.
2. Bailey RL, Gahche JJ, Lentino CV, et al. Dietary supplement use in the United States, 2003-2006. J Nutr 2011;141(2):261–6.
3. Andrès E, Loukili NH, Noel E, et al. Vitamin B12 (cobalamin) deficiency in elderly patients. CMAJ 2004;171(3):251.
4. Prentice A, Gail GR, Schoenmakers I. Vitamin D across the lifecycle: physiology and biomarkers. Am J Clin Nutr 2008;88(Suppl):500S–6S.
5. Larry JE. Vitamin nutrition in the elderly, geriatric nutrition: a comprehensive review. 2nd edition. New York: Raven Press; 1995.

6. Morley JE. Protein energy malnutrition in older subjects. Proc Nutr Soc 1998;57:587–92.
7. Sies H, Stahl W, Sundquist AR. Antioxidant functions of vitamins: vitamins E and C, β-carotene and other carotenoids. Ann N Y Acad Sci 1992;669:7–20.
8. Morley JE. The resurgence of free radicals. J Am Geriatr Soc 1992;40:1285–7.
9. Jacobs P, Wood L. Vitamin A. Dis Mon 2003;49(11):677–84.
10. The effect of vitamin E and beta-carotene on the incidence of lung cancer and other cancers in male smokers. The Alpha-Tocopherol, Beta-Carotene Cancer Prevention Study Group. N Engl J Med 1994;330:1029–35.
11. Omenn GS, Goodman GE, Thornquist MD, et al. Effects of combination of β-carotene and vitamin A on lung cancer and cardiovascular disease. N Engl J Med 1996;334:1150.
12. Virtamo J, Pietinen P, Huttunen JK, et al. Incidence of cancer and mortality following α-tocopherol and β-carotene supplementation: a postintervention follow-up. JAMA 2003;290(4):476–85.
13. Hennekens CH, Buring JE, Manson JE, et al. Lack of effect of long-term supplementation with beta carotene on the incidence of malignant neoplasms and cardiovascular disease. N Engl J Med 1996;334(18):1145.
14. Hunter DJ, Manson JE, Colditz GA, et al. A prospective study of the intake of vitamins C, E, and A and the risk of breast cancer. N Engl J Med 1993;329(4):234.
15. Zhang S, Hunter DJ, Forman MR, et al. Dietary carotenoids and vitamins A, C, and E and risk of breast cancer. J Natl Cancer Inst 1999;91(6):547.
16. Greenberg ER, Baron JA, Tosteson TD, et al. A clinical trial of antioxidant vitamins to prevent colorectal adenoma. Polyp Prevention Study Group. N Engl J Med 1994;331(3):141.
17. Christen WG, Manson JE, Glynn RJ, et al. A randomized trial of beta carotene and age-related cataract in US physicians. Arch Ophthalmol 2003;121:372.
18. Bressler N, Bressler S, Congdon N, et al. Age-Related Eye Disease Study Research Group. A randomized, placebo-controlled, clinical trial of high-dose supplementation with vitamins C and E, beta carotene, and zinc for age-related macular degeneration and vision loss: AREDS report no. 8. Arch Ophthalmol 2001;119(10):1417–36.
19. Chong EW, Wong TY, Kreis AJ, et al. Dietary antioxidants and primary prevention of age-related macular degeneration: systematic review and meta-analysis. BMJ 2007;335(7623):755.
20. Evans JR, Henshaw K. Antioxidant vitamin and mineral supplements for preventing age-related macular degeneration. Cochrane Database Syst Rev 2008;(1):CD000253.
21. Evans JR, Lawrenson JG. Antioxidant vitamin and mineral supplements for preventing age-related macular degeneration. Cochrane Database Syst Rev 2012;(6):CD000253.
22. Feskanich D, Singh V, Willett WC, et al. Vitamin A intake and hip fractures among post-menopausal women. JAMA 2002;287:47.
23. Michaelsson K, Lithell H, Vessby B, et al. Serum retinol levels and the risk of fracture. N Engl J Med 2003;348:287.
24. Olson RE. Vitamin deficiency, dependency and toxicity. In: Beers MH, Berkow R, editors. The Merck manual of diagnosis and therapy, Merck. NJ: Whitehouse Station; 1998. p. 32–51.
25. Reuben DB, Greendale GA, Harrison GG. Nutrition screening in older persons. J Am Geriatr Soc 1995;43:415–25.

26. Lippman SM, Klein EA, Goodman PJ, et al. Effect of selenium and vitamin E on risk of prostate cancer and other cancers: the Selenium and Vitamin E Cancer Prevention Trial (SELECT). JAMA 2009;301:39–51.
27. Gaziano JM, Glynn RJ, Christen WG, et al. Vitamins E and C in the prevention of prostate and total cancer in men: the Physicians' Health Study II randomized controlled trial. JAMA 2009;301:52–62.
28. Lin J, Cook NR, Albert C, et al. Vitamins C and E and beta carotene supplementation and cancer risk: a randomized controlled trial. J Natl Cancer Inst 2009;101: 14–23.
29. Stampfer MJ, Hennekens CH, Manson JE, et al. Vitamin E consumption and risk of coronary artery disease in women. N Engl J Med 1993;328(20):1444–9.
30. Rimm EB, Stampfer MJ, Ascherio A, et al. Vitamin E consumption and risk of coronary artery disease in men. N Engl J Med 1993;328(20):1450–6.
31. Lonn E, Bosch J, Yusuf S, et al. Effects of long-term vitamin E supplementation on cardiovascular events and cancer. JAMA 2005;293(11):1338–47.
32. Lonn EM, Yusuf S, Dzavik V, et al, SECURE Investigators. Effects of ramipril and vitamin E on atherosclerosis: the study to evaluate carotid and ultrasound changes in patients treated with ramipril and vitamin E (SECURE). Circulation 2001;103:919.
33. Leppala JM, Virtamo J, Fogelholm R, et al. Vitamin E and beta carotene supplementation in high risk for stroke: a subgroup analysis of the Alpha-Tocopherol, Beta-Carotene Cancer Prevention Study. Arch Neurol 2000;57:1503.
34. Engelhart MJ, Geerlings MI, Ruitenberg A, et al. Dietary intake of antioxidants and risk of Alzheimer disease. JAMA 2002;287:3223.
35. Morris MC, Evans DA, Bienias JL, et al. Dietary intake of antioxidant nutrients and the risk of incident Alzheimer disease in a biracial community study. JAMA 2002; 287:3230.
36. Sano M, Ernesto C, Thomas RG, et al, The Alzheimer's Disease Cooperative Study. A controlled trial of selegiline, alpha-tocopherol, or both as treatment for Alzheimer's disease. N Engl J Med 1997;336:1216.
37. Petersen RC, Thomas RG, Grundman M, et al, Alzheimer's Disease Cooperative Study Group. Vitamin E and donepezil for the treatment of mild cognitive impairment. N Engl J Med 2005;352(23):2379.
38. Kang JH, Cook N, Manson J, et al. A randomized trial of vitamin E supplementation and cognitive function in women. Arch Intern Med 2006;166:2462–8.
39. Miller ER III, Pastor-Barriuso R, Dalal D, et al. Meta-analysis: high-dosage vitamin E supplementation may increase all-cause mortality. Ann Intern Med 2005;142:37.
40. Jacob R. Vitamin C. In: Shils M, Olson J, Shike M, et al, editors. Modern nutrition in health and disease. Philadelphia: Lippincott; 2000. p. 467.
41. Johnson KA. Vitamin nutrition in the older adult. Clin Geriatr Med 2002;18:773–99.
42. McLaran CJ, Bett JH, Nye JA, et al. Congestive cardiomyopathy and haemochromatosis—rapid progression possibly accelerated by excessive ingestion of ascorbic acid. Aust N Z J Med 1982;12:187.
43. Vivekananthan DP, Penn MS, Sapp SK, et al. Use of antioxidant vitamins for the prevention of cardiovascular disease: meta-analysis of randomised trials. Lancet 2003;361:2017.
44. Ascherio A, Rimm EB, Hernan MA, et al. Relation of consumption of vitamin E, vitamin C and carotenoids to risk for stroke among men in the United States. Ann Intern Med 1999;130:963.
45. Hankinson SE, Stampfer MJ, Seddon JM, et al. Nutrient intake and cataract extraction in women: a prospective study. BMJ 1992;305:335.

46. Age-Related Eye Disease Study Research Group. A randomized, placebo-controlled, clinical trial of high-dose supplementation with vitamins C and E and β-carotene for age-related cataract and vision loss: AREDS Report No. 9. Arch Ophthalmol 2001;119:1439.
47. Hemilä H, Chalker E. Vitamin C for preventing and treating the common cold. Cochrane Database Syst Rev 2013;(1):CD000980.
48. Jackson RD, LaCroix AZ, Gass M, et al. Calcium plus vitamin D supplementation and the risk of fractures. N Engl J Med 2006;354:669–83.
49. Tang BM, Eslick GD, Nowson C, et al. Use of calcium or calcium in combination with vitamin D supplementation to prevent fractures and bone loss in people aged 50 years and older: a meta-analysis. Lancet 2007;370:657–66.
50. The DIPART (vitamin D Individual Patient Analysis of Randomized Trials) Group. Patient level pooled analysis of 68 500 patients from seven major vitamin D fracture trials in US and Europe. BMJ 2010;340:b5463.
51. Bischoff-Ferrari HA, Dawson-Hughes B, Staehelin HB, et al. Fall prevention with supplemental and active forms of vitamin D: a meta-analysis of randomized controlled trials. BMJ 2009;339:b3692.
52. Smith H, Anderson F, Raphael H, et al. Effect of annual vitamin D on fracture risk in elderly men and women: a population-based, randomized, double-blinded, placebo-controlled trial. Rheumatology 2007;46:1852–7.
53. Sanders KM, Stuart AI, Williamson EJ, et al. Annual high-dose oral vitamin D and falls and fractures in older women: a randomized controlled trial. JAMA 2010;303:1815–22.
54. Wang L, Song Y, Manson JE, et al. Circulating 25-hydroxy-vitamin D and risk of cardiovascular disease: a meta-analysis of prospective studies. Circ Cardiovasc Qual Outcomes 2012;5(6):819.
55. Pittas AG, Chung M, Trikalinos T, et al. Systematic review: vitamin D and cardiometabolic outcomes. Ann Intern Med 2010;152(5):307.
56. Scragg R, Sowers M, Bell C. Serum 25-hydroxyvitamin D, ethnicity, and blood pressure in the Third National Health and Nutrition Examination Survey. Am J Hypertens 2007;20(7):713.
57. Witham MD, Nadir MA, Struthers AD. Effect of vitamin D on blood pressure: a systematic review and meta-analysis. J Hypertens 2009;27(10):1948.
58. Giovannucci E. The epidemiology of vitamin D and cancer incidence and mortality: a review (United States). Cancer Causes Control 2005;16(2):83.
59. IARC. Vitamin D and Cancer. IARC Working Group Reports Vol. 5, International Agency for research on Cancer, Lyon. Available at: http://www.iarc.fr/en/publications/pdfs-online/wrk/wrk5/Report_VitD.pdf. Accessed November 22, 2014.
60. Wactawski-Wende J, Kotchen JM, Anderson GL, et al, Women's Health Initiative Investigators. Calcium plus vitamin D supplementation and the risk of colorectal cancer. N Engl J Med 2006;354(7):684.
61. Bjelakovic G, Gluud LL, Nikolova D, et al. Vitamin D supplementation for prevention of cancer in adults. Cochrane Database Syst Rev 2014;(6):CD007469.
62. Ozfirat Z, Chowdhury TA. Vitamin D deficiency and type 2 diabetes. Postgrad Med J 2010;86(1011):18.
63. Sollid ST, Hutchinson MY, Fuskevåg OM, et al. No effect of high-dose vitamin D supplementation on glycemic status or cardiovascular risk factors in subjects with prediabetes. Diabetes Care 2014;37(8):2123.
64. Giovannucci E, Stampfer MJ, Colditz GA, et al. Multivitamin use, folate, and colon cancer in women in the Nurses' Health Study. Ann Intern Med 1998;129(7):517.

65. Cole BF, Baron JA, Sandler RS, et al, Polyp Prevention Study Group. Folic acid for the prevention of colorectal adenomas: a randomized clinical trial. JAMA 2007; 297(21):2351.
66. Ebbing M, Bonaa KH, Nygård O, et al. Cancer incidence and mortality after treatment with folic acid and vitamin B12. JAMA 2009;302(19):2119.
67. Martí-Carvajal AJ, Solà I, Lathyris D, et al. Homocysteine lowering interventions for preventing cardiovascular events. Cochrane Database Syst Rev 2009;(4): CD006612.
68. Miller ER 3rd, Juraschek S, Pastor-Barriuso R, et al. Meta-analysis of folic acid supplementation trials on risk of cardiovascular disease and risk interaction with baseline homocysteine levels. Am J Cardiol 2010;106(4):517.
69. Jacobs P, Wood L. Vitamin B2. Dis Mon 2003;49(11):653–7.
70. Larsson SC, Orsini N, Wolk A. Vitamin B6 and risk of colorectal cancer: a meta-analysis of prospective studies. JAMA 2010;303(11):1077.
71. Zhang SM, Willett WC, Selhub J, et al. Plasma folate, vitamin B6, vitamin B12, homocysteine, and risk of breast cancer. J Natl Cancer Inst 2003;95(5):373.
72. Vogel T, Dali-Youcef N, Kaltenbach G, et al. Homocysteine, vitamin B12, folate and cognitive functions: a systematic and critical review of the literature. Int J Clin Pract 2009;63(7):1061–7.

Sarcopenia as the Biological Substrate of Physical Frailty

Francesco Landi, MD, PhD[a,*], Riccardo Calvani, PhD[a,1], Matteo Cesari, MD, PhD[b,1], Matteo Tosato, MD, PhD[a], Anna Maria Martone, MD[a], Roberto Bernabei, MD[a], Graziano Onder, MD, PhD[a], Emanuele Marzetti, MD, PhD[a]

KEYWORDS

• Skeletal muscle • Physical performance • Aging • Operationalization • Disability

KEY POINTS

- Skeletal muscle degeneration (sarcopenia) and decreasing homeostatic reserve (frailty) are hallmarks of the aging process, associated with several important health-related adverse events.
- Multiple operational definitions of physical frailty and sarcopenia have been produced, but wide consensus has not yet been reached.
- Physical function impairment represents the core feature shared by physical frailty and sarcopenia.
- The recognition of sarcopenia as the biological substrate of physical frailty allows framing an objectively measurable, standardized condition to be implemented in standard practice.

INTRODUCTION

Physical function decreases with aging, leading to a wide spectrum of negative outcomes, such as mobility disability, falls, social isolation, reduced quality of life,

This work was partly supported by a grant from the Innovative Medicines Initiative (IMI–JU 115621). The work was also supported by the "Centro Studi Achille e Linda Lorenzon" and a grant from the Italian Ministry of Education, Universities and Research (MIUR – linea D3.2, 2013).

No conflict of interest.

[a] Department of Geriatrics, Neurosciences and Orthopedics, Catholic University of the Sacred Heart, L.go A. Gemelli 8, Rome 00168, Italy; [b] Gérontopôle, University Hospital of Toulouse, 37 Allées Jules Guesde, Toulouse 31000, France

[1] These authors equally contributed to the article.

* Corresponding author. Centro Medicina dell'Invecchiamento (CEMI), Istituto di Medicina Interna e Geriatria, Università Cattolica del Sacro Cuore, Largo Agostino Gemelli 8, Roma 00168, Italy.

E-mail address: francesco.landi@rm.unicatt.it

Clin Geriatr Med 31 (2015) 367–374
http://dx.doi.org/10.1016/j.cger.2015.04.005 geriatric.theclinics.com
0749-0690/15/$ – see front matter

dependency, and institutionalization. The age-related loss of physical performance often results from multiple clinical and subclinical conditions.[1] Advancing age is linked with important changes in body composition, the most remarkable of which, sarcopenia, is a major cause of physical function decay, disability, and mortality.[2] After the age of 35 years, a healthy subject loses muscle mass at a rate of 1% to 2% per year in combination with a 1.5% annual decline in strength, which accelerates to around 3% per year after the age of 60.[3] As a consequence, the muscle cross-sectional area of the thigh decreases by about 40% between 20 and 60 years of age. The decline in fat-free mass is twice as great in men than in women, and is amplified in sedentary subjects relative to physically active peers.[3] While losing lean body mass, an average adult can be expected to gain approximately 0.50 kg of fat mass per year between the ages of 30 and 60.[4] This modification in body composition is frequently masked by unchanging body weight and can result in a disorder known as sarcopenic obesity, which greatly enhances the risk of adverse health outcomes.[5]

SARCOPENIA: FROM DEFINITION TO ASSESSMENT

The concept of sarcopenia is faced with growing frequency in research and clinical practice, not only in geriatric medicine but also in other specialties. Although sarcopenia is common and poses enormous individual and societal costs, there is not a widely accepted operational definition, nor a specific code in the International and Statistical Classification of Diseases and Health-related Problems, 10th edition (ICD-10), or specific treatment guidelines.[6,7]

The term sarcopenia derives from the Greek roots *sarx*, for flesh, and *penia*, for loss. It was originally used in 1988 at a meeting convened in Albuquerque, New Mexico, to refer to the most notable age-related change in body composition observed across species and associated with a number of negative health outcomes.[8–10] The proposal of using this term for indicating the skeletal muscle decline was indeed motivated by the attempt to stimulate research around one of the most evident and universal phenomena of aging.

From a practical point of view, sarcopenia may be considered an organ failure (muscle failure). It is typically chronic, although an acute onset is also possible (for example, during hospital stay). It is related, through physical frailty (PF), to the development of physical disability.

The European Working Group on Sarcopenia in Older People (EWGSOP)[11] proposed to articulate the detection of sarcopenia on the assessment of both muscle function (strength or performance) and muscle mass. In other words, the identification of sarcopenia is based on the presence of low muscle mass plus the concurrent presence of either low muscle strength or low physical performance. The recent reports by the Foundation of the National Institute of Health (FNIH) initiative have moved the field forward relative to existing operational definitions (including the one by the EWGSOP).[12] Different from previous recommendations that were largely based on experts' consensus, the major strength of the FNIH criteria can be found in the operationalization of the definition from the results of ad hoc analyses conducted in a large sample population (composed of multiple cohort studies).[12–14] It is also noteworthy that the FNIH reports tend to separate the qualitative from the quantitative domain of the sarcopenia definition, given the growing body of evidence reporting significant differences between muscle function and mass (especially in terms of predictive capacity and clinical relevance). Through the adoption of Classification and Regression Tree (CaRT) models, several muscle anthropometric variables were tested, and those that best predicted disability were identified.[15]

More in details, the FNIH project recommended two alternative gender-specific measures to define low muscle mass.[12] The first FNIH parameter (ie, appendicular lean mass [ALM]-to-body mass index [BMI] ratio, ALM_{BMI}) is the one recommended, while the second (ie, crude ALM) is proposed as an alternative. Given the relevance of the FNIH initiative and the adopted methodological approach, these definitions might be easily considered as the current best practice for defining low muscle mass in the elderly.

Physical Frailty as a Geriatric Syndrome

Based on a recent consensus definition, frailty has been defined as a geriatric "multidimensional syndrome characterized by decreased reserve and diminished resistance to stressors."[16] When frailty is envisioned as a predisability condition, it may then well serve as a target for preventive interventions. Unfortunately, although the theoretic concept of frailty is largely agreed upon, its translation into clinical practice still presents limitations, mainly because of the existence of multiple (and largely nonoverlapping) operational definitions.

According to the Survey of Health, Aging and Retirement in Europe (SHARE) study, the prevalence of prefrailty and frailty among 18,227 randomly selected community-dwellers aged 65 years or more across Europe was 42.3% (40.5%–44.1%) and 17.0% (15.3%–18.7%), respectively.[17] In the absence of targeted interventions, the progression of PF is marked by increased morbidity, disability, frequent and often inappropriate health care use, nursing home admission, and poor quality of life.[18] Identifying and contrasting PF are therefore of importance for hindering the evolution of the syndrome and preventing its negative consequences.[19] Indeed, once disability has developed, the restoration of a sufficient level of functioning is unlikely, particularly when the age of the subject, the degree of disability, or the disability's duration increases.

Unfortunately, to date, no health care programs or pharmacologic treatments are available for frail older subjects. This is mostly due to the lack of a unique definition of frailty. Such disagreement/controversy may easily be justified by the multidimensional and complex nature of the condition.[20] It is consequently not by accident that the syndrome is not yet nosographically contemplated (eg, it is not present in the ICD-10). The current gaps in knowledge are reflected by the lack of effective interventions (either pharmacologic or behavioral) against frailty. This barrier can be overcome by developing a robust theoretic framework of PF. This conceptualization should also expand the definition of the pathophysiologic and clinical bases of the condition to assist in the design of specific interventions aimed at restoring healthiness and postponing the development of adverse events (in particular, disability).

SARCOPENIA AND FRAILTY: DECONSTRUCTING THEIR INNER FOUNDATIONS

In the literature, different criteria have been validated to identify frail older subjects, which mainly refer to two conceptual models: the deficit accumulation approach proposed by Rockwood and colleagues[21] and the PF phenotype proposed by Fried and colleagues.[22] Both models have received empirical validation. To date, the frailty phenotype is probably the most widely used. It is mainly focused on exploring the physical domain of the frailty syndrome; thus it may present a better-characterized pathophysiologic background. The PF condition depicted by the frailty phenotype has shown to be predictive of major negative health-related outcomes, including mobility disability, disability for activities of daily living, institutionalization, and mortality.[23] At the same time, it cannot be ignored that the clinical picture of frailty (especially when focused on the physical domain) presents substantial overlap with that of sarcopenia.[7] In other words, sarcopenia might be considered both as the biological substrate for the development of PF and the physiopathologic pathway through which the negative health-related outcomes of PF ensue (**Fig. 1**).

Since the beginning, sarcopenia and frailty have been studied in parallel. Being organ-specific, sarcopenia was more frequently object of research in basic science, whereas the concept of frailty tended to be more easily applied in the clinical setting. Nevertheless, it was inevitable that the two would have sooner or later started converging, because both conditions deal with the common subclinical and clinical manifestations of aging. Unfortunately, the definition of a clear framework in which sarcopenia and frailty can be accommodated and studied has yet to come. One of the major issues in this context is indeed the long-lasting, tiring, and potentially pointless controversy about the causal relationship between the two. Determining whether frailty is caused by sarcopenia or sarcopenia is a clinical manifestation of frailty is consuming considerable efforts, but (from a very practical viewpoint) rather resembles the problem of the egg and the chicken.[24]

Deconstructing the inner foundations of these twin conditions and trying to focus on shared and clinical relevant features might represent a pragmatic means to solve the dilemma.

SARCOPENIA AND PHYSICAL FRAILTY: A NEW CONCEPTUAL MODEL OF DISEASE

For the construction of a practical conceptual model, sarcopenia may be considered the central element of the PF syndrome. By establishing a specific biological basis (ie, skeletal muscle decline) of PF, novel venues might be opened for the development of interventions aimed at slowing or reversing this disorder. In this respect, it is remarkable that all of the factors depicting PF and sarcopenia are quantifiable and measurable. Therefore, the implementation of this theoretic model will feasibly encourage

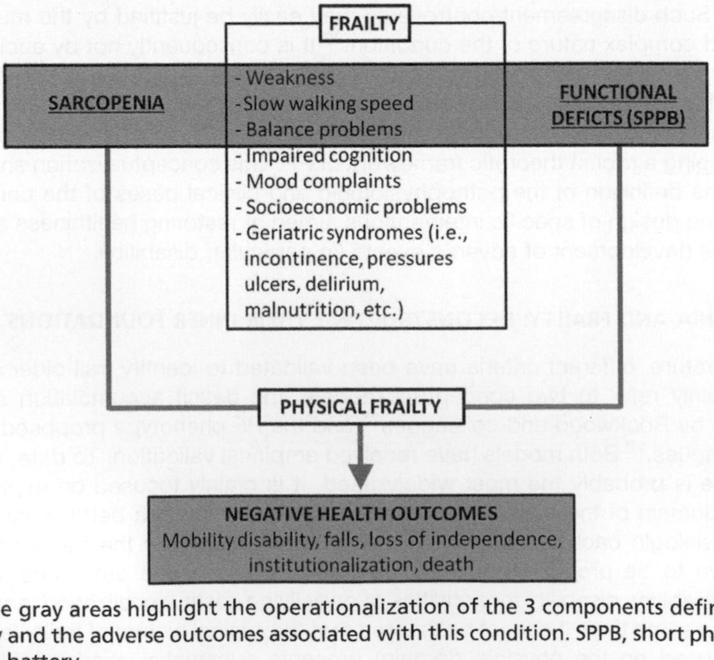

Fig. 1. The gray areas highlight the operationalization of the 3 components defining physical frailty and the adverse outcomes associated with this condition. SPPB, short physical performance battery.

important advancements over the traditional approaches to this syndrome by enabling the accurate operationalization of the disorder, a clear identification of the affected population, and the rapid translation of findings to the clinical settings. It is worth noting that such a conceptualization renders PF and sarcopenia comparable to other common geriatric conditions, with the great benefit of making the syndrome more easily acceptable by health care professionals, public health authorities, and regulatory bodies.

According to the proposed conceptual model, the PF and sarcopenia condition has a biological substrate at the level of muscle (ie, low muscle mass), easily and objectively measurable with available techniques (for example, by dual energy X-ray absorptiometry [DXA]) (**Table 1**). At the clinical level, the manifestations of the PF and sarcopenia condition, such as slow gait speed, impaired balance, and weakness, are also measureable in an objective manner with specific assessment scales, such as the Short Physical Performance Battery (SPPB).[25] This set of measurable biological substrate, measurable clinical manifestations, and measurable functional performance is similar to the diagnostic path that is usually performed for other common age-related degenerative conditions, such as congestive heart failure, chronic obstructive pulmonary disease, and peripheral artery disease (see **Table 1**). This eventually implies that older persons with PF and sarcopenia can easily be identified as those with target organ damage (ie, low muscle mass), specific clinical phenotype, and impaired physical performance.

Possible Strategies for Intervening Against Physical Frailty and Sarcopenia

The identification of sarcopenia as a major component of PF indicates that interventions specifically targeting the skeletal muscle may offer preventive and therapeutic advantages against frailty and its clinical correlates.[26] Observational studies and some randomized clinical trials (RCTs) have suggested a positive effect of regular physical activity (PA) and nutritional interventions on improving physical function and/or reducing symptoms of disability in healthy older individuals and those at risk for mobility disability. Unfortunately, definite evidence from high-quality, large-scale RCTs is still lacking. In this regard, it is important to recognize that short-term gains

Table 1
Conceptual framework of physical therapy and sarcopenia—resemblance to common conditions of advanced age

Condition	Measurable Biological Substrate	Measurable Clinical Manifestations	Measurable Function
CHF	Myocardial dysfunction (echocardiography)	• Shortness of breath • Fatigue	6-min walking test
COPD	Airways destructive changes (spirometry)	• Dyspnoea • Cough • Sputum	6-min walking test
PAD	Arterial stenosis (Doppler echocardiography)	• Intermittent claudication • Numbness • Ulcers	Treadmill walking distance
PF&S	Reduced muscle mass (DXA)	• Slow walking speed • Poor balance • Weakness	SPPB

Abbreviations: CHF, chronic heart failure; COPD, chronic obstructive pulmonary disease; DXA, dual energy X-ray absorptiometry; PAD, peripheral artery disease; PF&S, physical frailty and sarcopenia; SPPB, short physical performance battery.

in intermediate outcomes of PA programs, such as strength and aerobic capacity, are insufficient to prove that such programs can truly prevent frailty and disability.

To date, the largest and longest study in this field is the Lifestyle Interventions and Independence for Elders (LIFE) study,[27] a multicenter RCT conducted in the United States comparing a PA program with a successful aging educational program in 1635 sedentary and functionally limited older persons, over a follow-up period of approximately 3 years. The primary outcome of the study was the incidence of mobility disability as expressed by inability to walk 400 m. The PA program (intervention group) consisted of a combination of walking at moderate intensity, resistance exercises, balance, stretching, and behavioral counseling. The successful aging educational program (control group) consisted of health education seminars and upper extremity stretching exercises. Overall, the PA program reduced the incidence of major mobility disability over a mean follow-up period of 2.6 years, with largest benefits among participants with more severe functional impairment at baseline.[28] Secondary analyses in the LIFE pilot (LIFE-P) study database have also shown that the PA intervention is able to significantly reduce the prevalence of the frailty phenotype and the number of frailty criteria over 1 year of follow-up compared with controls. Remarkably, the beneficial effects of PA on the frailty score were, again, greater in participants showing a frailer status at baseline. Although the LIFE study was not designed to operationalize a conceptual model of PF nor was the PA intervention specifically targeted against PF and sarcopenia, these results suggest that behavioral interventions could positively impact PF and sarcopenia.

Apart from small RCTs, such as the FRAilty Screening and Intervention (FRASI) study,[29] no large-scale intervention studies explicitly targeting frail older subjects have been conducted. Given the complexity of the PF and sarcopenia syndrome, it is likely that the implementation of multicomponent interventions (MCIs), combining PA, nutrition and eventually drugs, might offer the greatest benefits in terms of prevention of incident disability and major negative health-related events. Notably, the implementation of preventive MCIs in older persons is particularly useful when dealing with age-related conditions requiring an immediate translation into clinical practice. Indeed, the simultaneous targeting of multiple and heterogeneous mechanisms underlying the disabling cascade may potentiate the intervention effects. Conversely, a monodimensional intervention may be insufficient at reversing the complex frailty status. At the same time, MCIs allow one to more easily translate the study results into clinical practice for the overall older population, thus reducing the well-known limited generalization of evidence-based studies. It is noteworthy that such multicomponent approaches resemble what is commonly done in usual clinical practice, in which the intervention is designed around the needs and resources of the individual.[26]

SUMMARY

The ongoing demographic transition is accompanied by substantial changes in medical needs and nosographic scenarios, which impose major actions against prevalent disabling conditions.[30] Frailty and sarcopenia are common, but not yet nosographically recognized geriatric syndromes that impact dramatically the health status of older adults. The lack of a widely accepted operationalization of these conditions hampers the design of effective preventive and therapeutic strategies, amplifying the socioeconomic burden associated with their detrimental consequences. Not surprisingly, the need of refining the assessments of sarcopenia and frailty is perceived as a high priority by the scientific and medical community as well as by health care authorities and regulators.

The core of the 2 conditions represented by the skeletal muscle decline in the absence of disability may optimally serve for (1) defining a novel target for interventions against disability, (2) facilitating the translation of the two conditions in the clinical arena and (3) providing an objective, standardized, and clinically relevant condition to be adopted by public health and regulatory agencies.

Such conceptualization might eventually encourage key stakeholders to join their efforts for approaching the sarcopenia and frailty conditions.[24]

REFERENCES

1. Cesari M, Vellas B, Gambassi G. The stress of aging. Exp Gerontol 2013;48:451–6.
2. Calvani R, Miccheli A, Landi F, et al. Current nutritional recommendations and novel dietary strategies to manage sarcopenia. J Frailty Aging 2013;2:38–53.
3. Hughes VA, Frontera WR, Roubenoff R, et al. Longitudinal changes in body composition in older men and women: role of body weight change and physical activity. Am J Clin Nutr 2002;76:473–81.
4. Forbes GB. Longitudinal changes in adult fat-free mass: influence of body weight. Am J Clin Nutr 1999;70:1025–31.
5. Waters DL, Baumgartner RN, Garry PJ, et al. Advantages of dietary, exercise-related, and therapeutic interventions to prevent and treat sarcopenia in adult patients: an update. Clin Interv Aging 2010;5:259–70.
6. Cruz-Jentoft AJ, Landi F. Sarcopenia. Clin Med 2014;14(2):183–6.
7. Cruz-Jentoft AJ, Landi F, Topinková E, et al. Understanding sarcopenia as a geriatric syndrome. Curr Opin Clin Nutr Metab Care 2010;13:1–7.
8. Landi F, Liperoti R, Fusco D, et al. Sarcopenia and mortality among older nursing home residents. J Am Med Dir Assoc 2012;13:121–6.
9. Landi F, Liperoti R, Russo A, et al. Sarcopenia as a risk factor for falls in elderly individuals: results from the ilSIRENTE study. Clin Nutr 2012;31:652–8.
10. Landi F, Cruz-Jentoft AJ, Liperoti R, et al. Sarcopenia and mortality risk in frail older persons aged 80 years and older: results from ilSIRENTE study. Age Ageing 2013;42:203–9.
11. Cruz-Jentoft AJ, Baeyens JP, Bauer JM, et al, European Working Group on Sarcopenia in Older People. Sarcopenia: European consensus on definition and diagnosis: report of the European working group on sarcopenia in older people. Age Ageing 2010;39:412–23.
12. Studenski SA, Peters KW, Alley DE, et al. The FNIH sarcopenia project: rationale, study description, conference recommendations, and final estimates. J Gerontol A Biol Sci Med Sci 2014;69:547–58.
13. Morley JE, Abbatecola AM, Argiles JM, et al. Sarcopenia with limited mobility: an international consensus. J Am Med Dir Assoc 2011;12:403–9.
14. Fielding RA, Vellas B, Evans WJ, et al. Sarcopenia: an undiagnosed condition in older adults. Current consensus definition: prevalence, etiology, and consequences. International working group on sarcopenia. J Am Med Dir Assoc 2011;12:249–56.
15. Cawthon PM, Peters KW, Shardell MD, et al. Cutpoints for low appendicular lean mass that identify older adults with clinically significant weakness. J Gerontol A Biol Sci Med Sci 2014;69:567–75.

16. Rodríguez-Mañas L, Féart C, Mann G, et al. Searching for an operational definition of frailty: a delphi method based consensus statement. The frailty operative definition—consensus conference project. J Gerontol A Biol Sci Med Sci 2012;68: 62–7.
17. Santos-Eggimann B, Cuenoud P, Spagnoli J, et al. Prevalence of frailty in middle-aged and older community-dwelling Europeans living in 10 countries. J Gerontol A Biol Sci Med Sci 2009;64:675–81.
18. Xue XL. The frailty syndrome: definition and natural history. Clin Geriat Med 2011; 27:1–15.
19. Morley JE, Vellas B, Abellan van Kan G, et al. Frailty consensus: a call to action. J Am Med Dir Assoc 2013;14:392–7.
20. Cesari M. The multidimentionality of frailty: many faces of one single dice. J Nutr Health Aging 2011;15:663–4.
21. Rockwood K, Song X, MacKnight C, et al. A global clinical measure of fitness and frailty in older people. CMAJ 2005;173(5):489–95.
22. Fried LP, Tangen CM, Walston J, et al. Frailty in older adults: evidence for a phenotype. J Gerontol A Biol Sci Med Sci 2001;56:M146–56.
23. Morley JE, Malmstrom TK, Miller DK. A simple frailty questionnaire (FRAIL) predicts outcomes in middle aged African Americans. J Nutr Health Aging 2012;16:601–8.
24. Cesari M, Landi F, Vellas B, et al. Sarcopenia and physical frailty: two sides of the same coin. Front Aging Neurosci 2014;6:192.
25. Guralnik JM, Simonsick EM, Ferrucci L, et al. A short physical performance battery assessing lower extremity function: association with self-reported disability and prediction of mortality and nursing home admission. J Gerontol 1994;49:M85–94.
26. Cruz-Jentoft AJ, Landi F, Schneider SM, et al. Prevalence of and interventions for sarcopenia in ageing adults: a systematic review. Report of the International Sarcopenia Initiative (EWGSOP and IWGS). Age Ageing 2014;43:748–59.
27. Fielding RA, Rejeski WJ, Blair S, et al, LIFE Research Group. The lifestyle interventions and Independence for elders study: design and methods. J Gerontol A Biol Sci Med Sci 2011;66(11):1226–37.
28. Pahor M, Guralnik JM, Ambrosius WT, et al. Effect of structured physical activity on prevention of major mobility disability in older adults: the LIFE study randomized clinical trial. JAMA 2014;311:2387–96.
29. Bandinelli S, Lauretani F, Boscherini V, et al. A randomized, controlled trial of disability prevention in frail older patients screened in primary care: the FRASI study. Design and baseline evaluation. Aging Clin Exp Res 2006;18(5):359–66.
30. Landi F, Martone AM, Calvani R, et al. Sarcopenia risk screening tool: a new strategy for clinical practice. J Am Med Dir Assoc 2014;15:613–4.

Frailty, Exercise and Nutrition

Jean-Pierre Michel, MD[a,*], Alfonso J. Cruz-Jentoft, MD[b], Tommy Cederholm, MD[c]

KEYWORDS

• Frailty • Sarcopenia • Physical exercise • Nutrition • Multicomponent intervention

KEY POINTS

- Age, genetics, epigenetics (nutrition, physical exercise), and environment play key roles in the frailty process.
- Frailty may be delayed or even reversed by physical exercise, with or without nutrition supplementation, or by targeted interventions on specific frailty components.
- A review of physical activities and nutrition interventions testified that sarcopenia, a major component of physical frailty, could be delayed or reversed.
- Multidomain interventions are promising. First results are encouraging, but the sole economic evaluation performed to date demonstrated the very high costs of such interventions.

Frailty is characterized by increased vulnerability to stressors that puts older subjects at risk of developing adverse outcomes, including hospitalization, disability, and mortality.[1,2] With population aging, frailty is becoming a silent epidemic, affecting older adults.[3] In the largest survey to date performed in Europe, namely the Survey of Health, Aging and Retirement in Europe (SHARE), a multidisciplinary, cross-national panel database of microdata on health, socioeconomic state, and social and family networks including more than 85,000 individuals aged 65 or over (approximately 150,000 interviews) from 19 countries across Europe and Israel,[4] the prevalence of frailty (using an adapted version of Fried's criteria of physical frailty[5]) reached 17%, varying from 5.8% in Switzerland to 27.3% in Spain. The prevalence of prefrailty was considerably higher, ranging from 34.6% in Germany to 50.9% in Spain.[6] In SHARE, mortality exponentially increased from robust to prefrail to frail subjects (**Fig. 1**).[7]

[a] Geriatric Department, Geneva University, 40 A Route de Malagnou, Geneva 1208, Switzerland; [b] Head of the Geriatric Department, University Hospital Ramón y Cajal, Carretera de Colmenar km 9, 1, Madrid 28034, Spain; [c] Department of Public Health and Caring Sciences, Clinical Nutrition and Metabolism, Uppsala University, Dag Hammarskjöldsv. 14B, Uppsala Science Park, 75185 Uppsala, Sweden
* Corresponding author.
E-mail address: jean-pierre.michel@unige.ch

Clin Geriatr Med 31 (2015) 375–387
http://dx.doi.org/10.1016/j.cger.2015.04.006 **geriatric.theclinics.com**
0749-0690/15/$ – see front matter

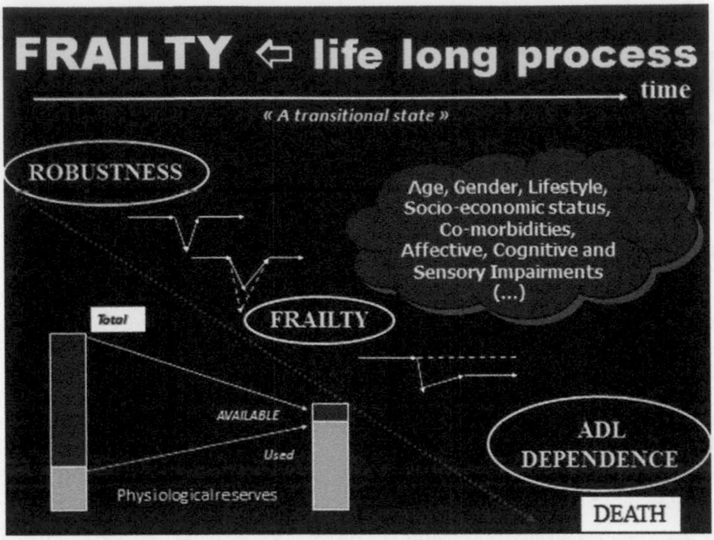

Fig. 1. Frailty is included in a transitional state between robustness, dependency, and death. ADL, activities of daily living.

Such data explain the urgent need to establish a universal definition of the frailty syndrome,[3] to detect prefrail individuals at an early stage in the community, and to implement effective prevention strategies.[8–10] Early intervention in frail individuals has the potential to retard or prevent disability, one of the key objectives of gerontology today.

The main components of the frailty phenotype as described by Fried and colleagues[5] are physical. Age, undernutrition, and sarcopenia play major roles in the vicious cycle of frailty,[11–13] explaining why various authors have proposed sarcopenia to be considered as the equivalent of physical frailty.[14–16] After the publication of the European consensus definition of sarcopenia,[17] a systematic review by an international working group of all published randomized trials (RCTs) showed that sarcopenia could be reversed, either by physical exercise, protein/amino acid diet interventions, or a combination thereof.[15] However, there again, the main problem with sarcopenia is its early detection, based on acknowledged criteria that need to be adapted to differences in the studied populations.[18–21]

In this rapidly evolving context, a major issue is linked to the fact that no consensus yet exists on how to identify prefrail and frail adults within the community, as recently stressed by the new British Geriatric Society guidelines.[22] The main purpose of the present article is to demonstrate that physical frailty, closely resembling sarcopenia, may be reversed by physical exercise, nutritional interventions, or a combination of the two. It should also be borne in mind that, beyond the physical features, the frailty syndrome also includes at least two other components, namely cognition and socioeconomic status.[23–25] Physical and cognitive frailty share some common pathogenetic pathways,[26] and consequently, certain interventions might impact both conditions.

This article first reports the spontaneous course of frailty conditions, and then focuses on randomized, controlled frailty interventions (such as physical exercise, nutrition, combined exercise plus nutrition, and multifactorial interventions) or metaanalysis in community-dwelling older adults or volunteers published in 2012, 2013, and 2014. The main take-home messages that emerge from recent literature are summarized.

DYNAMICS OF FRAILTY

The SHARE study[6] started in 2004 with a first epidemiologic survey using criteria adapted from Fried and colleagues namely shrinking, exhaustion, low physical activity, muscle weakness, and slow gait speed. This research was followed by 3 further surveys (waves) performed in 2006, 2009, and 2011.[4] Transitions between the different frailty states were analyzed. Observations from the first wave (2004) to the second (2006) included a follow-up of 14,448 European adults aged over age 65. In 2004, 52.1% of the population were not frail, 39.1% prefrail, and 8.8% frail. Two years later, without any known or programmed intervention, 22.1% had worsened, 61.8% had not changed, and 16.6% had improved their status.[27] Interestingly, among those whose status worsened, more than two-thirds moved from nonfrail in 2004 to prefrail at the next wave.[27] Over the same period, frail subjects were at increased risk of mobility disorders, comorbidities, and an inability to perform basic and instrumental activities of daily living (ADL; $P<.001$ for all).[28]

Between the second (2006) and the fourth (2011) waves, naturally occurring transitions were observed for 15,776 European adults.[29] The results presented in **Fig. 2**

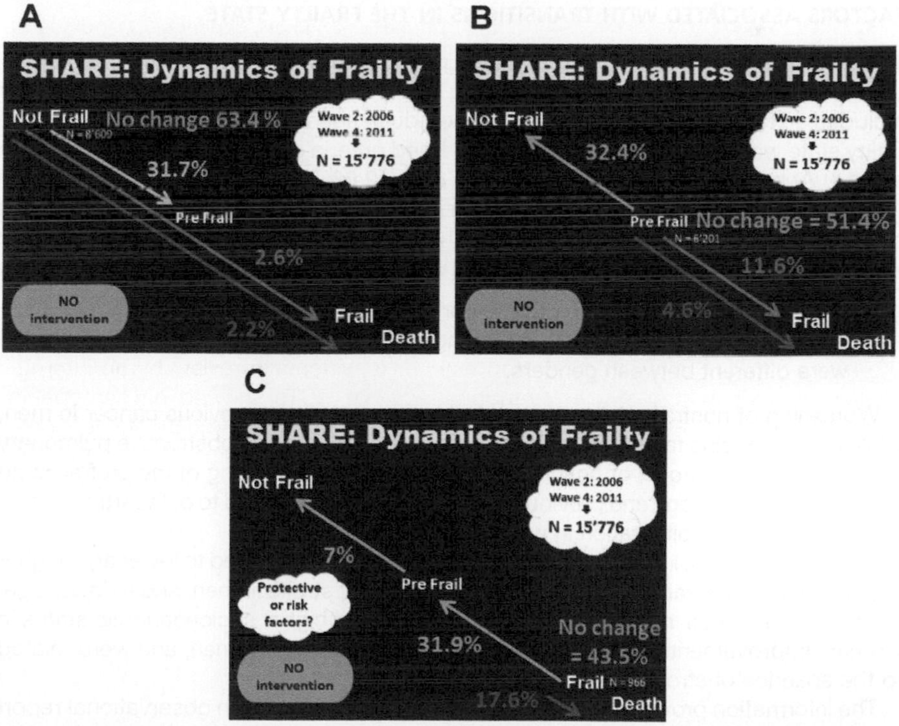

Fig. 2. (*A*) Natural transitions occurring from the not-frail state to other clinical conditions between the second (2006) and fourth (2011) waves of the SHARE study. (*B*) Natural transitions occurring from the prefrail state to other clinical conditions between the second (2006) and fourth (2011) waves of the SHARE study. (*C*) Natural transitions occurring from the frail state to other clinical conditions between the second (2006) and fourth (2011) waves of the SHARE study. (*Adapted from* Borrat-Besson C, Ryser VA, Wernli B. Transitions between frailty states – a European comparison. In: Börsch-Supan A, Brandt M, Litwin H, et al, editors. Active aging and solidarity between generations in Europe. Berlin: De Gruyter; 2013. p. 175–86.

confirm that the nonfrail or robust state deteriorates over time, as do the prefrail and frail states. Death is the unavoidable consequence of this temporal deterioration.

However, the most important and positive message to come out of these data is the reversibility of the prefrail state toward a robust state, observed in one-third of all individuals. A second optimistic message is that the frail state is also reversible in approximately one-third of the older adults studied, with transition toward the prefrail or even nonfrail state.

The Precipitating Events Project in the United States also confirmed that frailty among older persons is a dynamic process, characterized by frequent transitions between frailty states over time.[30] This study of 754 non–ADL-disabled community-living persons aged 70 years or older, using Fried's criteria, found that 57.6% of the participants had at least 1 transition between any 2 of the 3 frailty states over 54 months, with rates of 36.8%, 21.5%, and 9.2% for 1, 2, and 3 transitions, respectively. However, in this study, transitions to states of greater frailty were more common (rates of ≤43.3%) than transitions to states of lesser frailty (rates of ≤23.0%).

FACTORS ASSOCIATED WITH TRANSITIONS IN THE FRAILTY STATE

Two recent papers focused on identifying the factors that positively or negatively contribute to changing the frailty state. The most recent and informative study included 3018 community-dwelling Chinese adults aged over 65 years of age, whose frailty state was classified according to the Fried criteria on 2 visits performed 2 years apart.[31] At baseline, 850 (48.7%) men and 884 (52.6%) women were prefrail. Among these, 23.4% of men and 26.6% of women improved after 2 years, whereas 11.1% of men and 6.6% of women worsened.[31] Other important conclusions from this study were that there are important gender differences, namely:

- More men than women (*P*<.001) deteriorated into frailty
- Factors that accelerate the worsening or improvement of the functional state were different between genders.

Worsening of nonfrail adults was related to older age and previous cancer in men, while corresponding factors for women were older age, chronic obstructive pulmonary disease, previous stroke, or hospitalization. Moreover, worsening of the prefrail state was related to older age and previous hospitalization in men, and to osteoarthritis, previous stroke, or hospitalization in women.

On the other hand, improvement of the prefrail state was related to lower age, higher Mini Mental State Examination score, and absence of stroke in men, and to lower age, absence of diabetes, no previous hospitalization, and higher socioeconomic status in women. Improvements of the frail state were only observed in men, and were related to the absence of stroke.[31]

The information provided by this study is complemented by an observational report from the San Antonio Longitudinal Study of Aging on changes in frailty characteristics from 1992 through 1996 to 2000 through 2001 in a cohort of about 600 older Mexican Americans and European Americans (mean age of 70 years at inclusion).[32] In this study, the authors identified the following significant predictors of progression in any frailty characteristic:

- Diabetes with macrovascular complications (odds ratio [OR], 1.84; 95% CI, 1.02–3.33)
- Fewer years of education (OR, 0.96; 95% CI, 0.93–1.0).

Another important piece of information to come out of this study is that frail individuals were more likely to die than to remain frail. Indeed, death rates increased in line with poorer baseline frailty status, low performance-based measures, and low physical activity.[32] Taken together, this body of evidence indicates that frailty interventions could be important to facilitate frailty reversibility.[33,34]

In this article, only the results of randomized, controlled interventions in frail older adults published between 2012 and the end of 2014 are considered. Four types of interventions have been tested to date, namely physical exercise alone, nutritional supplements, a combination of physical exercise and nutrition, and multifactorial interventions.

PHYSICAL EXERCISE IN FRAIL ELDERS

Two metaanalyses of RCTs investigating the effects of exercise were published in 2012[35] and 2014.[36] The first metaanalysis included 8 RCTs, all published before 2010, and selected from among 146 trials.[35] The 8 trials investigated included 1068 frail participants selected according to predetermined Fried criteria (age range, 75.3–86.8 years) and randomly assigned to either the inactive control group or the exercise intervention group; that is, simple or comprehensive, lasting at least 60 minutes, twice a week with a follow-up of at least 8 months.[35] Frail individuals taking part in regular exercise showed improvements in several parameters, namely:

- Gait speed (evaluated in 4 trials, n = 459) increased by 0.07 m/s (95% CI, 0.02–0.11; $P = .005$)
- Berg Balance Scale score (fully evaluated in 3 trials, n = 356) improved by a weighted average of 1.69 (95% CI, 0.56–2.82)
- ADL performance improved; mean difference of 5.33 (95% CI, 1.01–9.64).

However, the exercise intervention had no significant effects on either the Timed Up & Go test (3 studies, n = 400) or quality of life (2 studies, n = 409 for the physical component and n = 187 for the mental health component).[35]

The second study, published in 2014, reports a systematic review and metaanalysis of 12 RCTs (published up to 2013), and compared multicomponent physical exercise programs with an inactive control group of community-dwelling older adults, defined as frail according to physical function and physical difficulties in ADL.[36] Again, physical exercise programs (at least 45 minutes twice a week with follow-up from 6 months to 2 years) had a positive impact on several variables, namely:

- Normal gait speed (mean improvement 0.07 m/s; [95% CI, 0.04–0.09])
- Fast gait speed (mean improvement 0.08 m/s; [95% CI, 0.02–0.14])
- Short physical performance battery scores (mean improvement, 2.18; [95% CI, 1.56–2.80]).

Conversely, results were inconclusive for endurance outcomes, and no consistent effect was observed either on balance or ADL functional mobility. Moreover, the evidence comparing different modalities of exercise was scarce and heterogeneous.[36]

Based on these recent data, it seems clear that physical exercise programs can delay or reverse the prefrailty or frailty states. It is important to mention that the RCTs included in the two metaanalyses are totally different, but still yielded similar positive results. However, the exercise programs and the length of follow-up varied considerably from 1 RCT to another, precluding any specific recommendations regarding the type, duration, or frequency of physical exercise.

The largest study on the impact of increased physical activity in older subjects is the Lifestyle Interventions and Independence for Elders (LIFE) trial,[37] which randomized subjects to a physical activity intervention versus successful aging education. This study recently published data on frailty obtained from 424 community-dwelling persons (mean age, 76.8 years) with a sedentary lifestyle and at risk of mobility disability.[38] The prevalence of frailty at 12 months was significantly lower in the intervention group (10%) compared with the control group (19.1%). The number of frailty criteria was also reduced in frail and multimorbid subjects.

NUTRITION IN FRAIL ELDERS

RCTs of nutritional interventions in frail individuals remain scarce, although the role of undernutrition in the frailty process is well-established.[11] Thus, the preventive impact of protein-energy supplementation in frail older adults remains to be proven.

One recent RCT on this indication included 87 frail community-based adults (usual gait speed <0.6 m/s; Mini Nutritional Assessment <24; mean age, 78 years) with low socioeconomic status.[39] The intervention group received two 200-mL cans of a liquid formula providing 400 kcal, 25 g protein, 9.4 g essential amino acids, and 400 mL water per day for 12 weeks, and its impact was compared with a control group who received no supplementation.[39]

- Overall physical functioning did not change in the control group but improved by 5.9% in the intervention group.
- The short physical performance battery score declined by 12.5% in the control group, but remained stable in the intervention group.
- Gait speed decreased in both groups, but to a greater extent in the control group (11.3%) compared with the nutrition intervention group (1.1%).
- The Timed Up and Go score decreased by 11.3% in the controls, whereas it increased by 7.2% in the nutrition group.
- There were no changes in either group in hand grip strength or 1-legged standing performance.[39]

A second RCT assessed the impact of 24 weeks of dietary protein supplementation on muscle mass, strength, and physical performance in 65 frail older people, defined by Fried's criteria.[40]

- Skeletal muscle mass and type I and II muscle fibers did not change in any group.
- Muscle strength (leg extension strength) increased from 57.5 to 68.5 kg in the protein group compared with an increase from 57.5 to 63.5 kg in the placebo group.
- Physical performance (measured with the short physical performance battery) improved significantly from 8.9 to 10.0 of 12 points in the protein group, but did not change in the placebo group (from 7.8 to 7.9 points).[40]

Overall, these RCTs favor protein supplementation, which seems to delay or improve the frailty process, as measured by physical performance.

COMBINATION OF PHYSICAL EXERCISE AND NUTRITION INTERVENTIONS

Tieland and colleagues[41] explored the role of protein supplementation to augment the skeletal muscle response to resistance-type exercise training in older frail individuals.

They carried out an RCT among 62 frail older subjects (mean age, 78 years) who participated in a progressive resistance-type exercise training program (2 sessions per week for 24 weeks) during which they were supplemented twice daily with either protein (2 $\times$ 15 g) or a placebo.[41] The authors observed the following:

- Lean body mass increased from 47.2 kg to 48.5 kg in the protein group and did not change in the placebo group (from 45.7 kg to 45.4 kg)
- Muscle strength and physical performance improved significantly in both groups, with no added effect of dietary protein supplementation.[41]

MULTIFACTORIAL RANDOMIZED, CONTROLLED INTERVENTIONS

Numerous multidomain interventions are ongoing,[42–45] including a very ambitious international European trial,[46] but very few have been published to date. Nevertheless, an Australian team has published a series of interesting reports based on a single-center RCT on 241 frail elders (mean age, 83 years; 68% women) selected in accordance with the Fried criteria.[47,48] The intervention comprised a multifactorial interdisciplinary program targeted to address different features of frailty (including physiotherapy twice weekly, and support from a psychologist and health care worker), whereas the control group received usual care. Two hundred sixteen participants (90%) completed the 12-month study.[48] The authors observed a significantly lesser prevalence of frailty (the primary endpoint) in the intervention group compared with controls (absolute difference, 14.7%; 95% CI, 2.4–27; $P = .02$; number needed to treat, 6.8). No changes were observed between the 2 groups in terms of Barthel index, depressive symptoms, or health-related quality of life.[48]

The second report to come out of this RCT included 241 frail, community-dwelling older people without severe cognitive impairment, recently discharged from an elderly care and rehabilitation service, and was focused on:

- Gait speed
- Life Space Assessment (mobility-related disability, measured in terms of restriction on participation and limitation of activity; participation was evaluated in terms of satisfaction and performance during the preceding month)[49,50]
- Goal Attainment Scale (achievement of individualized mobility-related participation goals)[49,51]
- Reintegration to Normal Living Index (self-report measures of participation across multiple areas of life, using 9 of the 11 original criteria[49,52]).

At 12 months, the results were quite surprising in the intervention group:

- No change in gait speed
- Significant improvement in Life Space Assessment ($P<.004$)
- Significant improvement in Goal Attainment Scale ($P<.005$)
- Significant improvement in the Reintegration to Normal Living Index ($P<.0001$).[49,53]

These positive results demonstrated that focused intervention on specific frailty components yielded significant improvements, using different tools and scales that were probably closer to the patients' daily life and well-being.

Finally, these authors also performed a health-economic evaluation[54] based on the incremental cost-effectiveness ratios showing the following:

- In the overall population, the 12-month cost for 1 extra person to transition out of frailty was US$14,114 (2011 prices)

- In the subgroup of "very frail" participants, the 12-month cost for 1 extra person to transition out of frailty was US$36,525 (2011 prices).[54]

The conclusion of the Australian authors of this positive, multidomain intervention study in frail, community-dwelling older adults is that the intervention program yielded good value for money, and was particularly cost saving and cost effective in the population of very frail participants.[54]

Still, this is a fairly costly investment for any country to bear. Thus, there is a need to define simple selection processes (eg, phone selection of frail patients) and interventions (eg, e-health). A pilot study performed in Taiwan used the Chinese version of the Canadian Study of Health and Aging Clinical Frailty Scale Telephone Version (CCSHA_CFS_TV) to select frail older community dwelling participants for inclusion in the study protocol.[55] The authors reported that the CCSHA_CS_TV was an easy way to perform first stage screening of prefrail or frail older adults, with the following advantages[56]:

- It can be administrated quickly by telephone (in <2 minutes) by interviewers without formal training in geriatrics
- It has satisfactory interrater reliability and criterion validity
- The exclusion criteria are easily identified: communication barriers, too healthy or too ill, or institutionalized.

A second round of selection was subsequently performed in a local community hospital. The trial included 117 community-dwelling older adults and 122 controls selected after the phone interview (mean age, 71.4 ± 3.7 years; 59% females). Using a 2-by-2 factorial design, the participants, whose baseline characteristics were comparable, were randomly assigned to one of 3 groups:

- Exercise and nutrition (n = 55), whereby subjects received nutrition consultation/advice and 1 hour of aerobic and endurance exercise 3 times per week for 12 months.
- Problem solving therapy (PST; n = 57), comprising 6 sessions of psychological support over 3 months.
- Controls (non-exercise and nutrition [n = 62] or non-PST [n = 60]).

The global results of this study were mixed as the subjects randomized to exercise and nutrition showed:

- An improvement of their frailty state compared with non-exercise and nutrition subjects (45% vs 27%; adjusted P = .008) at 3 months, but this improvement was no longer significant at 6 or 12 months
- An increase of serum 25(OH) vitamin D level (4.9 ± 7.7 vs 1.2 ± 5.4; P = .006) at 6 months
- A lower percentage of osteopenia (74% vs 89% P = .042) at 12 months.

In the PST group, subjects showed an improvement of their frailty state at 6 months (2.7 ± 6.1 vs 0.2 ± 6.7; P = .035) and less deterioration at 12 months (−3.5 ± 9.7 vs −7.1 ± 8.7; P = .036) compared with non-PST subjects.

A recent, innovative Dutch study tested an e-health–based intervention model for frail community living elders.[57] A highly comprehensive protocol was established based on a community network including other old patients, their informal and formal care givers (general practitioners and general practitioners' assistants, as well as community health care professionals). The intervention group (n = 290) used a health and welfare portal (called ZWIP) allowing online health communications, and 392 patients were allocated to the control group. The most important findings from this study were that:

- Only 26.2% of the participants in the intervention group actively used the online portal during the 12 months protocol
- The participants yielded a nonsignificant improvement in basic and instrumental ADL.[57]

These somewhat disappointing results obtained from a rural population in the Netherlands deserve some consideration. Perhaps the same protocol used in another context with patients more aware and adept in using modern technology might have yielded different results.

TAKE HOME MESSAGES

- Age, genetics, epigenetics (nutrition, physical exercise), and environment play key roles in the frailty process.
- The most important message concerning intervention in frail elders is that frailty may be delayed or even reversed by physical exercise, with or without nutrition supplementation, or by targeted interventions on specific frailty components. This positive conclusion is provocative, because it is becoming urgent to identify the most effective and least costly interventions to be applied to the whole aging population. Effective screening of frailty and early targeted intervention is considered key in optimizing the care of frail populations at risk by health care authorities in Europe.[58]
- A recent review of isolated or combined physical activities and nutrition interventions testified that sarcopenia, which is a major component of physical frailty, could be delayed or reversed.[14] However, it is not yet well established whether the frailty syndrome, which is much more complex than the sarcopenia syndrome, can also be delayed or reversed.

The review of the RCTs published between 2012 and 2014 on this topic does not show convincing effects of either isolated physical activities or isolated protein supplementation. The combined intervention comprising nutrition plus exercise seems to be the mainstay of frailty treatment.

- The field of multidomain interventions is promising. First results are encouraging, but the sole economic evaluation performed to date demonstrated the very high costs of such interventions.

Indeed, these findings will stimulate more research, which is surely needed to help us face the global frailty challenge as quickly as possible.

The scientific community needs to urgently address several issues:

- Define the most simple and accurate criteria to select older, community-dwelling, prefrail adults
- Implement long-term, accurately powered randomized controlled interventions
- Choose adequate tools to accurately evaluate the most relevant and important concerns of the patients, and not only scientific measurements
- Use modern technology to facilitate the entire research procedure, and empower older adults to use this technology for research purposes, but also for their own comfort and security in daily life
- Evaluate carefully the best way of increasing the cost-effectiveness of such interventions.

The twenty-first century of geriatric medicine lies ahead, and preventing sarcopenia, frailty, and their dramatic consequences is a crucial and urgent need.

ACKNOWLEDGMENTS

The authors thank Fiona Ecarnot (EA3920, University Hospital Besancon, France) for her assistance in the preparation of this manuscript.

REFERENCES

1. Clegg A, Young J, Iliffe S, et al. Frailty in elderly people. Lancet 2013;381:752–62.
2. Strandberg TE, Pitkala KH, Tilvis RS. Frailty in older people. Eur Geriatr Med 2011;2:344–55.
3. Cherubini A, Demougeot L, Cruz Jentoft A, et al. Validation of the gérontopôle frailty screening tool to detect frailty in primary care. Eur Geriatr Med 2015, in press.
4. Borsch-Supan A, Brandt M, Hunkler C, et al. Data resource profile: the survey of health, ageing and retirement in Europe (SHARE). Int J Epidemiol 2013;42: 992–1001.
5. Fried LP, Tangen CM, Walston J, et al. Frailty in older adults: evidence for a phenotype. J Gerontol A Biol Sci Med Sci 2001;56:M146–56.
6. Santos-Eggimann B, Cuenoud P, Spagnoli J, et al. Prevalence of frailty in middle-aged and older community-dwelling Europeans living in 10 countries. J Gerontol A Biol Sci Med Sci 2009;64:675–81.
7. Romero-Ortuno R. The frailty instrument of the survey of health, ageing and retirement in Europe (SHARE-FI) predicts mortality beyond age, comorbidities, disability, self-rated health, education and depression. Eur Geriatr Med 2011;2: 323–6.
8. Morley JE. Frailty: a time for action. Eur Geriatr Med 2013;4:215–6.
9. Morley JE, Vellas B, van Kan GA, et al. Frailty consensus: a call to action. J Am Med Dir Assoc 2013;14:392–7.
10. Vellas B, Balardy L, Gillette-Guyonnet S, et al. Looking for frailty in community-dwelling older persons: the Gerontopole Frailty Screening Tool (GFST). J Nutr Health Aging 2013;17:629–31.
11. Fried LP, Hadley EC, Walston JD, et al. From bedside to bench: research agenda for frailty. Sci Aging Knowledge Environ 2005;2005:pe24.
12. Boirie Y, Morio B, Caumon E, et al. Nutrition and protein energy homeostasis in elderly. Mech Ageing Dev 2014;136–137:76–84.
13. Xue QL, Bandeen-Roche K, Varadhan R, et al. Initial manifestations of frailty criteria and the development of frailty phenotype in the Women's Health and Aging Study II. J Gerontol A Biol Sci Med Sci 2008;63:984–90.
14. Sieber C. Sarcopenia and frailty. In: Crutz-Jentoft AJ, Morley JE, editors. Sarcopenia. Chichester; West Sussex (United Kingdom): Wiley-Blackwell; 2012.
15. Cruz-Jentoft AJ, Landi F, Schneider SM, et al. Prevalence of and interventions for sarcopenia in ageing adults: a systematic review. Report of the International Sarcopenia Initiative (EWGSOP and IWGS). Age Ageing 2014;43:748–59.
16. Cesari M, Landi F, Vellas B, et al. Sarcopenia and physical frailty: two sides of the same coin. Front Aging Neurosci 2014;6:192.
17. Cruz-Jentoft AJ, Baeyens JP, Bauer JM, et al. Sarcopenia: European consensus on definition and diagnosis: report of the European Working Group on Sarcopenia in Older People. Age Ageing 2010;39:412–23.

18. Morley JE, Abbatecola AM, Argiles JM, et al. Sarcopenia with limited mobility: an international consensus. J Am Med Dir Assoc 2011;12:403–9.
19. Chen LK, Liu LK, Woo J, et al. Sarcopenia in Asia: consensus report of the Asian Working Group for Sarcopenia. J Am Med Dir Assoc 2014;15:95–101.
20. Cruz-Jentoft AJ, Triana FC, Gomez-Cabrera MC, et al. The emergent role of sarcopenia: preliminary report of the observatory of Sarcopenia of the Spanish Society of Geriatrics and Gerontology. Rev Esp Geriatr Gerontol 2011;46:100–10 [in Spanish].
21. Michel JP. Sarcopenia: there is a need for some steps forward. J Am Med Dir Assoc 2014;15:379–80.
22. Turner G, Clegg A. Best practice guidelines for the management of frailty: a British Geriatrics Society, Age UK and Royal College of General Practitioners report. Age Ageing 2014;43:744–7.
23. Kelaiditi E, Cesari M, Canevelli M, et al. Cognitive frailty: rational and definition from an (I.A.N.A./I.A.G.G.) international consensus group. J Nutr Health Aging 2013;17:726–34.
24. Guessous I, Luthi JC, Bowling CB, et al. Prevalence of frailty indicators and association with socioeconomic status in middle-aged and older adults in a Swiss region with universal health insurance coverage: a population-based cross-sectional study. J Aging Res 2014;2014:198603.
25. Dent E, Hoogendijk EO. Psychosocial factors modify the association of frailty with adverse outcomes: a prospective study of hospitalised older people. BMC Geriatr 2014;14:108.
26. Halil M, Cemal Kizilarslanoglu M, Kuyumcu ME, et al. Cognitive aspects of frailty: mechanisms behind the link between frailty and cognitive impairment. J Nutr Health Aging 2015;19(3):276–83.
27. Etman A, Burdorf A, Van der Cammen TJ, et al. Socio-demographic determinants of worsening in frailty among community-dwelling older people in 11 European countries. J Epidemiol Community Health 2012;66:1116–21.
28. Macklai NS, Spagnoli J, Junod J, et al. Prospective association of the SHARE-operationalized frailty phenotype with adverse health outcomes: evidence from 60+ community-dwelling Europeans living in 11 countries. BMC Geriatr 2013;13:3.
29. Borrat-Besson C, Ryser VA, Wernli B. Transitions between frailty states – a European comparison. In: Börsch-Supan A, Brandt M, Litwin H, et al, editors. Active ageing and solidarity between generations in Europe. Berlin: De Gruyter; 2013. p. 175–86. Available at: http://www.degruyter.com/view/books/9783110295467/9783110295467.175/9783110295467.175.xml. Accessed May 5, 2015.
30. Gill TM, Gahbauer EA, Allore HG, et al. Transitions between frailty states among community-living older persons. Arch Intern Med 2006;166:418–23.
31. Lee JS, Auyeung TW, Leung J, et al. Transitions in frailty states among community-living older adults and their associated factors. J Am Med Dir Assoc 2014;15(4):281–6.
32. Espinoza SE, Jung I, Hazuda H. Frailty transitions in the San Antonio longitudinal study of aging. J Am Geriatr Soc 2012;60:652–60.
33. Binder EF, Schechtman KB, Ehsani AA, et al. Effects of exercise training on frailty in community-dwelling older adults: results of a randomized, controlled trial. J Am Geriatr Soc 2002;50:1921–8.
34. Gill TM, Baker DI, Gottschalk M, et al. A program to prevent functional decline in physically frail, elderly persons who live at home. N Engl J Med 2002;347:1068–74.

35. Chou CH, Hwang CL, Wu YT. Effect of exercise on physical function, daily living activities, and quality of life in the frail older adults: a meta-analysis. Arch Phys Med Rehabil 2012;93:237–44.
36. Gine-Garriga M, Roque-Figuls M, Coll-Planas L, et al. Physical exercise interventions for improving performance-based measures of physical function in community-dwelling, frail older adults: a systematic review and meta-analysis. Arch Phys Med Rehabil 2014;95:753–69.e3.
37. Pahor M, Guralnik JM, Ambrosius WT, et al. Effect of structured physical activity on prevention of major mobility disability in older adults: the LIFE study randomized clinical trial. JAMA 2014;311:2387–96.
38. Cesari M, Vellas B, Hsu FC, et al. A physical activity intervention to treat the frailty syndrome in older persons-results from the LIFE-P study. J Gerontol A Biol Sci Med Sci 2015;70(2):216–22.
39. Kim CO, Lee KR. Preventive effect of protein-energy supplementation on the functional decline of frail older adults with low socioeconomic status: a community-based randomized controlled study. J Gerontol A Biol Sci Med Sci 2013;68:309–16.
40. Tieland M, Borgonjen-Van den Berg KJ, van Loon LJ, et al. Dietary protein intake in community-dwelling, frail, and institutionalized elderly people: scope for improvement. Eur J Nutr 2012;51:173–9.
41. Tieland M, Dirks ML, van der Zwaluw N, et al. Protein supplementation increases muscle mass gain during prolonged resistance-type exercise training in frail elderly people: a randomized, double-blind, placebo-controlled trial. J Am Med Dir Assoc 2012;13:713–9.
42. Spoorenberg SL, Uittenbroek RJ, Middel B, et al. Embrace, a model for integrated elderly care: study protocol of a randomized controlled trial on the effectiveness regarding patient outcomes, service use, costs, and quality of care. BMC Geriatr 2013;13:62.
43. Cesari M, Demougeot L, Boccalon H, et al. The Multidomain Intervention to preveNt disability in ElDers (MINDED) project: rationale and study design of a pilot study. Contemp Clin Trials 2014;38:145–54.
44. Rodriguez-Manas L, Bayer AJ, Kelly M, et al. An evaluation of the effectiveness of a multi-modal intervention in frail and pre-frail older people with type 2 diabetes–the MID-Frail study: study protocol for a randomised controlled trial. Trials 2014;15:34.
45. Romera L, Orfila F, Segura JM, et al. Effectiveness of a primary care based multifactorial intervention to improve frailty parameters in the elderly: a randomised clinical trial: rationale and study design. BMC Geriatr 2014;14:125.
46. Bernabei R, Vellas B. Sarcopenia and physical frailty in older people: multicomponent treatment strategies. [serial on the Internet]. 2014. Available at: www.mysprintt.eu. Accessed May 05, 2015.
47. Fairhall N, Aggar C, Kurrle SE, et al. Frailty intervention trial (FIT). BMC Geriatr 2008;8:27.
48. Cameron ID, Fairhall N, Langron C, et al. A multifactorial interdisciplinary intervention reduces frailty in older people: randomized trial. BMC Med 2013;11:65.
49. Fairhall N, Sherrington C, Kurrle SE, et al. Effect of a multifactorial interdisciplinary intervention on mobility-related disability in frail older people: randomised controlled trial. BMC Med 2012;10:120.
50. Baker PS, Bodner EV, Allman RM. Measuring life-space mobility in community-dwelling older adults. J Am Geriatr Soc 2003;51:1610–4.

51. Rockwood K, Stolee P, Fox RA. Use of goal attainment scaling in measuring clinically important change in the frail elderly. J Clin Epidemiol 1993;46:1113–8.
52. Wood-Dauphinee SL, Opzoomer MA, Williams JI, et al. Assessment of global function: the reintegration to normal living index. Arch Phys Med Rehabil 1988; 69:583–90.
53. Fairhall N, Sherrington C, Lord SR, et al. Effect of a multifactorial, interdisciplinary intervention on risk factors for falls and fall rate in frail older people: a randomised controlled trial. Age Ageing 2014;43:616–22.
54. Fairhall N, Sherrington C, Kurrle SE, et al. Economic evaluation of a multifactorial, interdisciplinary intervention versus usual care to reduce frailty in frail older people. J Am Med Dir Assoc 2015;16:41–8.
55. Chan DC, Tsou HH, Yang RS, et al. A pilot randomized controlled trial to improve geriatric frailty. BMC Geriatr 2012;12:58.
56. Rockwood K, Song X, MacKnight C, et al. A global clinical measure of fitness and frailty in elderly people. CMAJ 2005;173:489–95.
57. Makai P, Perry M, Robben SH, et al. Evaluation of an eHealth intervention in chronic care for frail older people: why adherence is the first target. J Med Internet Res 2014;16:e156.
58. De Manuel Keenoy E, David M, Mora J, et al. Activation of stratification strategies and results of the interventions on frail patients of healthcare services (ASSEHS) DG Sanco project No. 2013 12 04. Eur Geriatr Med 2014;5:342–6.

Dehydration, Hypernatremia, and Hyponatremia

John E. Morley, MB, BCh

KEYWORDS

• Dehydration • Hypernatremia • Hyponatremia • Osmolality • SIADH • Thirst
• Electrolytes • Aging

KEY POINTS

- Old persons have a poor thirst sensation putting them at major risk for dehydration.
- Subcutaneous infusions (hypodermaclysis) are an excellent way to treat dehydration in older persons.
- Hyponatremia caused by the syndrome of inappropriate antidiuretic hormone is very common in older persons.

Even small alterations in serum sodium are associated with poor outcomes.[1,2] With aging there is a marked reduction in body water from 70% of weight in infants to 50% in older persons.[3] Water plays several key roles in maintaining bodily function, such as waste product removal; a medium for transport of nutrients, hormones, and gases; thermoregulation; providing an environment conducive to chemical reactions; and as a shock absorber in bones.[4] The concept of aging being associated with relative dehydration is not a new one, being first recognized by the ancient Greeks: old age is "dried olive branch" (Homer), "dry and cold" (Aristotle), and a "decline in…body water" (Galen).[5] With aging, occurrences of hypernatremia and hyponatremia are very common, with elevated plasma tonicity occurring in up to a half of older persons[6] and half of persons in nursing homes developing at least one episode of hyponatremia.[7] In young persons, serum osmolality is tightly regulated between 135 and 142 nmol/L; when the system fails to do this, cells are exposed to hypotonic or hypertonic stress. In the hospital, increased mortality is seen when the sodium is greater than 142 mmol/L or less than 138 mmol/L.[8] Frail older persons are particularly at risk for developing electrolyte abnormalities.[9–12] Electrolyte abnormalities are a major

Divisions of Geriatric Medicine and Endocrinology, Saint Louis University School of Medicine, 1402 South Grand Boulevard, M238, St Louis, MO 63104, USA
E-mail address: morley@slu.edu

Clin Geriatr Med 31 (2015) 389–399
http://dx.doi.org/10.1016/j.cger.2015.04.007

cause of sarcopenia and functional decline.[13–17] Cognitive impairment is also common in persons with electrolyte abnormalities.[18,19] Falls are a common presentation of older persons with either hyponatremia or hypernatremia.[20–23]

DEHYDRATION

Dehydration is defined as a decline in total body water and can be caused by either water loss (hypertonic) or salt loss (hypotonic). Water loss dehydration is caused by a failure to ingest adequate fluid or excess water loss through the kidneys (eg, hyperglycemia), and salt loss dehydration is caused by water and salt loss. With aging, older persons have a decline in thirst caused by alterations in opioid, relaxin, and angiotensin II actions.[24–26] The major causes of salt loss dehydration are vomiting, diarrhea, sweating, hyperventilation, bleeding, exercise, and increased renal losses.

The primary test for dehydration is serum or plasma osmolality measured by freezing point (milliosmoles per kilogram). Calculated serum osmolarity includes urea, which moves freely between cells and the extracellular environment and, thus, is not an ideal measure. Calculated serum tonicity (effective osmolarity) is a better measure:

$$\text{Effective osmolarity} = 2Na + 2K = \text{glucose (in millimoles per liter)}$$

where *Na* is sodium and *K* is potassium.

Recently, it was shown that salivary osmolality detects water and sodium loss dehydration.[27] If repeated, this would make it the diagnostic test of choice for dehydration. Total body water by deuterium dilution would be considered the gold standard but has not been used clinically. The accuracy of bioelectrical impedance to examine acute changes in hydration status has been questioned and should not be used.[28–30] An elevated serum sodium associated with a low urine sodium is a reasonable proxy for serum osmolality.

Although physicians classically use a blood urea nitrogen (BUN) to creatinine ratio greater than 20 as an indicator of dehydration, this is not recommended.[4] Besides dehydration, the BUN/creatinine ratio is elevated by bleeding, heart and renal failure, increased protein intake, glucocorticoids, and glycyrrhizic acid (licorice). In addition, sarcopenia (aging muscle loss) results in a reduction in serum creatinine, thus increasing the BUN/creatinine ratio.[31,32]

In younger persons, the clinical diagnosis of dehydration has been considered the appropriate approach to diagnosis. However, in older persons, clinical symptoms and signs do not have adequate specificity or sensitivity. Skin turgor is generally a poor sign in older persons because of inelasticity of aging skin. If skin turgor is to be used in older persons, it should be done on the forehead. A moist oral mucosa tends to rule out dehydration, but a dry oral mucosa is very common in older persons. Orthostasis and tachycardia occur in most persons with dehydration but have many other causes.[33] Dry axilla has been shown to have an 82% specificity but a much lesser sensitivity for dehydration.[34] Delirium is commonly caused by dehydration in older persons.[35–38] Mild dehydration causes mild cognitive impairment and may result in anxiety, headache, agitated behavior, lethargy, delusions, and hallucinations in persons with underlying dementia.[18,39,40] A rapid weight loss over 1 to 2 weeks should always lead to consideration of dehydration as well as other causes of anorexia and weight loss.[41–43] Dark urine color has been found to be suggestive of dehydration.[44,45] Urine color has a reasonable correlation with specific gravity. However, Rowat and colleagues[46] could find no correlation between urine color or specific gravity and dehydration.

A dehydration checklist consisting of 31 items has been developed, but this complex diagnostic still tends to overidentify persons at risk for dehydration.[47] The Dehydration Council[4] developed a simple screening tool for dehydration risk:

- *D*iuretics
- *E*nd of life
- *H*igh fever
- *Y*ellow urine turns dark
- *D*izziness (orthostasis)
- *R*educed oral intake
- *A*xilla dry
- *T*achycardia
- *I*ncontinence (fear of)
- *O*ral problems (sippers)
- *N*eurologic impairment (confusion)
- *S*unken eyes

CYCORE (University of California, San Diego, CA) is a cyber infrastructure developed to use mobile sensors to allow older persons at risk of dehydration to be monitored at home.[48]

An algorithmic approach to diagnosing dehydration is given in **Fig. 1**.

To prevent dehydration, the recommendations for daily total water intake vary from 2.0 L/d (Europe) to 2.8 L/d (Australia) for women and 2.5 L/d to 3.7 L/d for men. This recommendation corresponds to 1.0 to 2.2 L of fluid intake daily for women and 1.2 to 3.0 L/d for men. The rest of the water comes from ingested food. Although fluid intake charts are recommended in hospitals and nursing homes, most of these are not completed or are inaccurate.[49,50]

Many approaches have been developed to try and prevent dehydration in older persons, especially in hospitals and nursing homes. A key is to enhance education for nursing staff, nursing aides, and physicians.[51,52] Physicians have been shown to make mistakes in the diagnosis in at least a third of the time.[53]

In the community, it is particularly important to increase the awareness that hot weather can play a role in producing dehydration. For persons older than 75 years, the in-hospital mortality rate for dehydration is about 10%.[54,55] Persons with respiratory diseases, heart failure, and renal failure are particularly susceptible to heat waves.[56] Providing increased awareness of the need to avoid going out in the heat, making available safe air conditioned areas, and stressing the importance of increasing fluid intake are important public health measures for community elders during heat waves.[57]

Institutional responses to preventing dehydration include providing straws and modified cups to improve fluid intake; being aware of the problems of giving adequate fluids in persons on texture-modified diets[58] and thickened liquids[59]; offering fluids regularly, using a snack and hydration cart[60]; providing preferred beverages; offering frozen juice bars; involving family; verbal prompting and assisting with drinking[61]; and "water clubs."[62] A systematic review by Bunn and colleagues[63] pointed out that although there are many strategies to increase fluid intake, there is little evidence base for the strategies.

When a person is clearly dehydrated, oral replacement is often inadequate. The formula for calculating fluid deficit is

$$\text{Fluid deficit} = \left[\frac{\text{serum Na}}{140}\right] \times \text{usual body weight(kg)} \times 0.5 - (\text{body weight/kg} \times 0.5)$$

where *Na* is sodium.

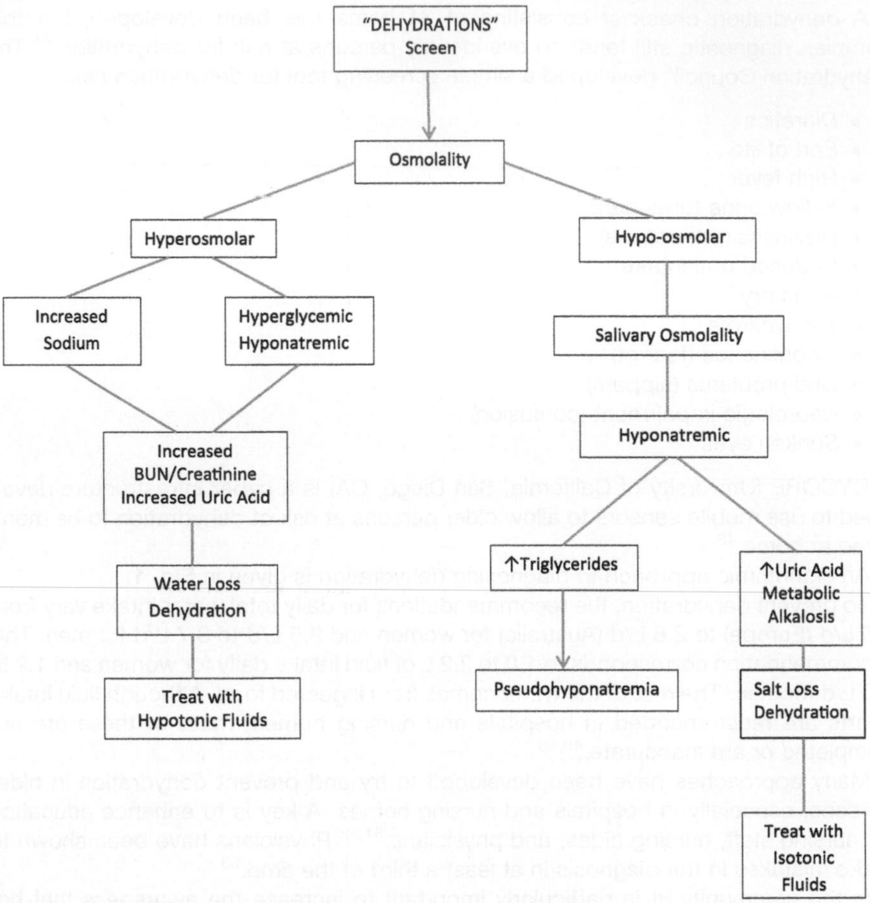

Fig. 1. Algorithmic approach to the diagnosis of dehydration (total body loss).

In addition to the fluid deficit, one must add insensible fluid loss (~500 mL/d) and urine loss. Insensible fluid loss is greatly increased with fever and in persons who have increased respiratory effort.

While in the hospital, most fluid is replaced intravenously; obtaining and maintaining a vein is often difficult at home or in institutions. In these cases, subcutaneous infusion (hypodermoclysis) is much easier.[64–66] It is easier to initiate and maintain and is less likely to be associated with bacteremia. It rarely leads to volume overload. It is extremely cost-effective. Despite these advantages, it is underused in nursing homes.

Dehydration is a relatively common problem with poor outcomes in older persons. It is particularly common in persons with dementia[67] and those receiving end-of-life care.[68] Clinical diagnosis is difficult, requiring the health professional to have a high index of suspicion for obtaining osmolality to make the diagnosis. For institutions, it is important that a dehydration prevention plan is practiced. Subcutaneous infusions are underutilized to treat dehydration. Dehydration has been identified as an important quality-of-life issue for which more research is needed in the nursing home.[69–71]

HYPONATREMIA

Hyponatremia is defined as a serum sodium level of less than 135 mM. Hyponatremia occurs more commonly in older persons than in younger persons. Hyponatremia occurs in 10.0% to 14.5% of community-dwelling older persons.[72–74] In these older persons, severe hyponatremia (<125 mmol/L) occurs in 1%. In nursing home residents, the incidence of hyponatremia is 22% to 25%.[7] When followed for a year, 53% of nursing home residents had at least one episode of hyponatremia. The incidence of mild hyponatremia on geriatric wards was 22.2% and 4.5% for severe hyponatremia.[74] Older women are more likely to develop hyponatremia than older men. In hospitals, older persons with a serum sodium less than 130 mmol/L had a mortality of 38% within 3 months of admission.[75] Severe hyponatremia is associated with a prolonged hospital stay. In the Rotterdam community study of older persons, those with hyponatremia had a 5-fold greater mortality.[76]

Hyponatremia is associated with delirium and mild cognitive impairment,[60,77,78] mobility and balance impairment[79,80] and falls.[81–83] Persons with hyponatremia have poorer performance on all the tests used for comprehensive geriatric assessment.[84] Hyponatremia is also a marker of frailty.[85–87] Very low sodium levels also can result in seizures.[88]

Hyponatremia is associated with an increase in bone fractures. In the Osteoporotic Fracture in Men (MrOs) study, hyponatremia doubled the risk of spine and hip fractures.[89] Cervellin and colleagues[90] found a similar high association of hyponatremia in persons with hip fracture presenting to the emergency department. Four other studies have also found fractures to be associated with hyponatremia.[76,91–93]

Persons with hyponatremia also have a lower bone mineral density at the hip.[94–96] An animal study demonstrated that hyponatremia increased bone resorption.[94] Persons with hyponatremia have a longer hospital stay following hip fracture.[97] Persons with hyponatremia have elevated arginine vasopressin (AVP) levels. AVP receptors are present on both osteoblasts and osteoclasts.[98] In rodents, AVP enhanced osteoclastic activity and reduced osteoblastic activity. Antagonists to or genetic deletion of AVP receptors resulted in increased bone mass.

There are numerous causes of hyponatremia. They can be euvolemic, hypovolemic, or hypervolemic:

Euvolemic hyponatremia

- Syndrome of inappropriate antidiuretic hormone
  - Intracranial pathologic conditions (stroke, tumors, infection, total brain injury)
  - Tumors (eg, lung, pancreas)
  - Lung diseases
  - Surgical procedures
  - Acquired immune deficiency syndrome
  - Pain
  - Nephrogenic (renal V2 receptor abnormality)
  - Mutation of transient receptor potential vanilloid type 4 (TRP V4) results in decreased ability to sense hypo-osmolality
- Hypothyroidism

Hypervolemic hyponatremia

- Congestive heart failure
- Cirrhosis
- Renal disease
- Exercise-induced hyponatremia (with excess fluid ingestion during exercise)

Hypovolemic hyponatremia

- Vomiting and diarrhea
- Diuretics
- Addison disease (adrenal insufficiency)
- Diabetes mellitus

In addition, a variety of drugs can lead to hyponatremia. Besides diuretics the most common drugs causing hyponatremia are antidepressants, especially selective serotonin reuptake inhibitors, amitriptyline, antipsychotic drugs, proton pump inhibitors, rivastigmine, antiepileptic drugs, opiates, and ciprofloxacin.[74] Excess drinking of beer can lead to hyponatremia caused by beer potomania.

Treatment of hyponatremia begins with treating the underlying cause. For persons with hypovolemic hyponatremia, the primary treatment is to increase the salt level using intravenous administration of normal (0.9%) saline. In persons with euvolemic hyponatremia, fluid restriction is the primary treatment. When the sodium level is less than 120 mmol/L, hypertonic (3%) saline is used to prevent long-term damage to the brain. Care needs to be taken not to correct the sodium too quickly as this can result in osmotic demyelination.[99] The rate of correction of osmolality should be between 8 and 12 mmol/L in the first 24 hours and no more than 18 mmol/L in the first 48 hours.[100]

Vaptans are nonpeptide AVP antagonists. By inhibiting the action of AVP on the kidney, they increase free water excretion.[101] The 2 approved vaptans are conivaptan, which can be used short-term intravenously in the hospital, and tolvaptan, which is oral and is approved for up to a 30-day use. Vaptans are used for either hypovolemic or euvolemic hyponatremia. Tolvaptan is safe and corrects sodium to normal.[102] It should be avoided in liver disease. For older persons, tolvaptan is more pleasant than water restriction. Only one small study found a clinical benefit, which was enhancement of gait function.[79] Vaptans are expensive, making their utility, given the paucity of data showing clinical improvement, questionable in most cases.

SUMMARY

Either an increase or a decrease in sodium levels is very common in older persons. Both increase mortality in older persons and are associated with delirium and falls. Awareness of the causes of these electrolyte disturbances can lead to appropriate prevention of severe disturbances. Treatment includes treating the underlying cause as well as returning sodium to the normal range.

REFERENCES

1. El-Sharkawy AM, Sahota P, Maughan RJ, et al. The pathophysiology of fluid and electrolyte balance in the older adult surgical patient. Clin Nutr 2014;33:6–13.
2. Hooper L, Bunn D, Jimoh FO, et al. Water-loss dehydration and aging. Mech Ageing Dev 2014;136–137:50–8.
3. Olde-Rikkert MG, Deurenberg P, Jansen RW, et al. Validation of multi-frequency bioelectrical impedance analysis in detecting changes in fluid balance of geriatric patients. J Am Geriatr Soc 1997;45:1345–51.
4. Thomas DR, Cote TR, Lawhorne L, et al. Understanding clinical dehydration and its treatment. J Am Med Dir Assoc 2008;9:292–301.
5. Morley JE. A brief history of geriatrics. J Gerontol A Biol Sci Med Sci 2004; 59(11):1132–52.
6. Stookey JD, Pieper CF, Cohen HJ. Is the prevalence of dehydration among community-dwelling older adults really low? Informing current debate over the

fluid recommendation for adults aged 70+ years. Public Health Nutr 2005;8(8): 1275–85.
7. Miller M, Morley JE, Rubenstein LZ. Hyponatremia in a nursing home population. J Am Geriatr Soc 1995;43(12):1410–3.
8. Wald R, Jaber BL, Price LL, et al. Impact of hospital-associated hyponatremia on selected outcomes. Arch Intern Med 2010;170(3):294–302.
9. Feinsod FM, Levenson SA, Rapp K, et al. Dehydration in frail, older residents in long-term care facilities. J Am Med Dir Assoc 2004;5(2 Suppl):S35–41.
10. Morley JE. Frailty screening comes of age. J Nutr Health Aging 2014;18(5): 453–4.
11. Malmstrom TK, Miller DK, Morley JE. A comparison of four frailty models. J Am Geriatr Soc 2014;62(4):721–6.
12. Morley JE. Frailty, falls, and fractures. J Am Med Dir Assoc 2013;14(3):149–51.
13. Miller M. Hyponatremia: age-related risk factors and therapy decisions. Geriatric 1998;53(7):32–3, 37–8, 41–2 passim.
14. Landi F, Martone AM, Calvani R, et al. Sarcopenia risk screening tool: a new strategy for clinical practice. J Am Med Dir Assoc 2014;15(9):613–4.
15. Michel JP. Sarcopenia: there is a need for some steps forward. J Am Med Dir Assoc 2014;15(6):379–80.
16. Rossi AP, Fantin F, Micciolo R, et al. Identifying sarcopenia in acute care setting patients. J Am Med Dir Assoc 2014;15(4):303.e7–12.
17. Woo J, Leung J, Morley JE. Defining sarcopenia in terms of incident adverse outcomes. J Am Med Dir Assoc 2015;16(3):247–52.
18. Wilson MM, Morley JE. Impaired cognitive function and mental performance in mild dehydration. Eur J Clin Nutr 2003;57(Suppl 2):S24–9.
19. Morley JE. Mild cognitive impairment—a treatable condition. J Am Med Dir Assoc 2014;15(1):1–5.
20. Büchele G, Becker C, Cameron ID, et al. Predictors of serious consequences of falls in residential aged care: analysis of more than 70,000 falls from residents of Bavarian nursing homes. J Am Med Dir Assoc 2014;15:559–63.
21. Wehling M. Morbus diureticus in the elderly: epidemic overuse of a widely applied group of drugs. J Am Med Dir Assoc 2013;14(6):437–42.
22. Morley JE, Rolland Y, Tolson D, et al. Increasing awareness of the factors producing falls: the mini falls assessment. J Am Med Dir Assoc 2012;13(2):87–90.
23. Rochat S, Monod S, Seematter-Bagnoud L, et al. Fallers in postacute rehabilitation have worse functional recovery and increased health services use. J Am Med Dir Assoc 2013;14:832–6.
24. Phillips PA, Bretherton M, Johnston CI, et al. Reduced osmotic thirst in healthy elderly men. Am J Physiol 1991;261(1 Pt 2):R166–71.
25. Silver AJ, Morley JE. Role of the opioid system in the hypodipsia associated with aging. J Am Geriatr Soc 1992;40(6):556–60.
26. Silver AJ, Flood JF, Morley JE. Effect of aging on fluid ingestion in mice. J Gerontol 1991;46:B117–21.
27. Fortes MB, Owen JA, Raymond-Barker P, et al. Is this elderly patient dehydrated? Diagnostic accuracy of hydration assessment using physical signs, urine, and saliva markers. J Am Med Dir Assoc 2014;16(3):221–8.
28. Kafri MW, Myint PK, Doherty D, et al. The diagnostic accuracy of multi-frequency bioelectrical impedance analysis in diagnosing dehydration after stroke. Med Sci Monit 2013;19:548–70.
29. Silver AJ, Guillen CP, Kahl MJ, et al. Effect of aging on body fat. J Am Geriatr Soc 1993;41:211–3.

30. Buffa R, Mereu RM, Putzu PF, et al. Bioelectrical impedance vector analysis detects low body cell mass and dehydration in patients with Alzheimer's disease. J Nutr Health Aging 2010;14(10):823–7.
31. Messinger-Rapport BJ, Gammack JK, Thomas DR, et al. Clinical update on nursing home medicine: 2013. J Am Med Dir Assoc 2013;14(12):860–76.
32. Soenen S, Chapman IM. Body weight, anorexia, and undernutrition in older people. J Am Med Dir Assoc 2013;14:642–8.
33. Iwanczyk L, Weintraub NT, Rubenstein LZ. Orthostatic hypotension in the nursing home setting. J Am Med Dir Assoc 2006;7(3):163–7.
34. Eaton D, Bannister P, Mulley GP, et al. Axillary sweating in clinical assessment of dehydration in ill elderly patients. BMJ 1994;308(6939):1271.
35. Flaherty JH, Morley JE. Delirium in the nursing home. J Am Med Dir Assoc 2013; 14:632–4.
36. Rudolph JL, Archambault E, Kelly B, VA Boston Delirium Task Force. A delirium risk modification program is associated with hospital outcomes. J Am Med Dir Assoc 2014;15:957.
37. Eeles E, Rockwood K. Delirium in the long-term care setting: clinical and research challenges. J Am Med Dir Assoc 2008;9:157–61.
38. Morandi A, Davis D, Fick DM, et al. Delirium superimposed on dementia strongly predicts worse outcomes in older rehabilitation inpatients. J Am Med Dir Assoc 2014;15:349–54.
39. Messinger-Rapport BJ, Gammack JK, Little MO, et al. Clinical update on nursing home medicine: 2014. J Am Med Dir Assoc 2014;15(11):786–801.
40. Flaherty JH, Morley JE. Delirium: a call to improve current standards of care. J Gerontol A Biol Sci Med Sci 2004;59(4):341–3.
41. Morley JE. Weight loss in the nursing home. J Am Med Dir Assoc 2007;8(4): 201–4.
42. Morley JE. Undernutrition in older adults. Fam Pract 2012;29(Suppl 1):i89–93.
43. Morley JE. Undernutrition: a major problem in nursing homes. J Am Med Dir Assoc 2011;12(4):243–6.
44. Wakefield BJ, Mentes J, Holman JE, et al. Postadmission dehydration: risk factors, indicators, and outcomes. Rehabil Nurs 2009;34(5):209–16.
45. Armstrong LE, Johnson EC, McKenzie AL, et al. Interpreting common hydration biomarkers on the basis of solute and water excretion. Eur J Clin Nutr 2013; 67(3):249–53.
46. Rowat A, Smith L, Graham C, et al. A pilot study to assess if urine specific gravity and urine colour charts are useful indicators of dehydration in acute stroke patients. J Adv Nurs 2011;67(9):1976–83.
47. Mentes JC, Wang J. Measuring risk for dehydration in nursing home residents: evaluation of the dehydration risk appraisal checklist. Res Gerontol Nurs 2011; 4(2):148–56.
48. Peterson SK, Shinn EH, Basen-Engquist K, et al. Identifying early dehydration risk with home-based sensors during radiation treatment: a feasibility study on patients with head and neck cancer. J Natl Cancer Inst Monogr 2013;47:162–8.
49. Scales K, Pilsworth J. The important of fluid balance in clinical practice. Nurs Stand 2008;22:50–7.
50. Kayser-Jones J, Schell ES, Porter C, et al. Factors contributing to dehydration in nursing homes: inadequate staffing and lack of professional supervision. J Am Geriatr Soc 1999;47:1187–94.
51. Keller H, Beck AM, Namasivayam A, International-Dining in Nursing home Experts (I-DINE). Improving food and fluid intake for older adults living in

long-term care: a research agenda. J Am Med Dir Assoc 2014;15(2): 93–100.
52. Crecelius C. Dehydration: myth and reality. J Am Med Dir Assoc 2008;9(5): 287–8.
53. Thomas DR, Tariq SH, Makhdomm S, et al. Physician misdiagnosis of dehydration in older adults. J Am Med Dir Assoc 2004;5(2 Suppl):S30–4.
54. Kettaneh A, Fardet L, Mario N, et al. The 2003 heat wave in France: hydration status changes in older inpatients. Eur J Epidemiol 2010;25(7): 517–24.
55. Rikkert MG, Melis RJ, Claassen JA. Heat waves and dehydration in the elderly. BMJ 2009;339:b2663.
56. Khalaj B, Lloyd G, Sheppeard V, et al. The health impacts of heat waves in five regions of New South Wales, Australia: a case-only analysis. Int Arch Occup Environ Health 2010;83(7):833–42.
57. Abdallah L, Remington R, Houde S, et al. Dehydration reduction in community-dwelling older adults: perspectives of community health care providers. Res Gerontol Nurs 2009;2:49–57.
58. Bannerman E, McDermott K. Dietary and fluid intakes of older adults in care homes requiring a texture modified diet: the role of snacks. J Am Med Dir Assoc 2011;12:234–9.
59. McGrail A, Kelchner LN. Adequate oral fluid intake in hospitalized stroke patients: does viscosity matter? Rehabil Nurs 2012;37(5):252–7.
60. Morley JE. Clinical practice in nursing homes as a key for progress. J Nutr Health Aging 2010;14(7):586–93.
61. Godfry H, Cloete J, Dymond E, et al. An exploration of the hydration care of older people: a qualitative study. Int J Nurs Stud 2012;49:1200–11.
62. Gleibs IH, Haslam C, Haslam SA, et al. Water clubs in residential care: is it water or the club that enhances health and well-being? Psychol Health 2011;26(10): 1361–77.
63. Bunn D, Jimoh F, Wilsher SH, et al. Increasing fluid intake and reducing dehydration risk in older people living in long-term care: a systematic review. J Am Med Dir Assoc 2015;16:101–13.
64. Garrett D. Use of hypodermoclysis to manage dehydration. How can subcutaneous fluids be used in the care of older people who are dehydrated? Nurs Older People 2013;25(4):12.
65. Dolamore MJ. The use of hypodermoclysis without hyaluronidase. J Am Med Dir Assoc 2009;10(1):75 [author reply: 75–6].
66. Gabriel J. Subcutaneous fluid administration and the hydration of older people. Br J Nurs 2014;23(14):S10 S12–4.
67. Vandervoort A, Van den Block L, van der Steen JT, et al. Nursing home residents dying with dementia in Flanders, Belgium: a nationwide postmortem study on clinical characteristics and quality of dying. J Am Med Dir Assoc 2013;14(7): 485–92.
68. Toot S, Devine M, Akporobaro A, et al. Causes of hospital admission for people with dementia: a systematic review and meta-analysis. J Am Med Dir Assoc 2013;14:463–70.
69. Morley JE, Caplan G, Cesari M, et al. International survey of nursing home research priorities. J Am Med Dir Assoc 2014;15:309–12.
70. Rolland Y, Tolson D, Morley JE, et al. The International Association of Gerontology and Geriatrics (IAGG) nursing home initiative. J Am Med Dir Assoc 2014;15:307–8.

71. Tolson D, Rolland Y, Andrieu S, et al. The International Association of Gerontology and Geriatrics: a global agenda for clinical research and quality of care in nursing homes. J Am Med Dir Assoc 2011;12(3):184–9.
72. Miller M, Hecker MS, Friedlander DA, et al. Apparent idiopathic hyponatremia in an ambulatory geriatric population. J Am Geriatr Soc 1996;44(4):404–8.
73. Caird FI, Andrews GR, Kennedy RD. Effect of posture on blood pressure in the elderly. Br Heart J 1973;35(5):527–30.
74. Mannesse CK, Vondeling AM, van Marum RJ, et al. Prevalence of hyponatremia on geriatric wards compared to other settings over four decades: a systematic review. Ageing Res Rev 2013;12:165–73.
75. Frenkel WN, van den Blom BJ, van Munster BC, et al. The association between serum sodium levels at time of admission and mortality and morbidity in acutely admitted elderly patients: a prospective cohort study. J Am Geriatr Soc 2010;58: 2227–8.
76. Hoorn EJ, Rivadeneira F, van Meurs JB, et al. Mild hyponatremia as a risk factor for fractures; the Rotterdam Study. J Bone Miner Res 2011;26(8):1822–8.
77. Miller M. Hyponatremia and arginine vasopressin dysregulation: mechanisms, clinical consequences, and management. J Am Geriatr Soc 2006;54(2):345–53.
78. Croxson M, Lucas J, Bagg W. Diluting delirium. N Z Med J 2005;118(1222): U1661.
79. Renneboog B, Musch W, Vandemergel X, et al. Mild chronic hyponatremia is associated with falls, unsteadiness, and attention deficits. Am J Med 2006; 119(1):71.
80. Lange-Asschenfeldt C, Kojda G, Cordes J, et al. Epidemiology, symptoms, and treatment characteristics of hyponatremic psychiatric inpatients. J Clin Psychopharmacol 2013;33:799–805.
81. Bun S, Serby MJ, Friedmann P. Psychotropic medication use, hyponatremia, and falls in an inpatient population. J Clin Psychopharm 2011;31:395–7.
82. Ahamed S, Anpalahan M, Savvas S, et al. Hyponatraemia in older medical patients: implications for falls and adverse outcomes of hospitalisation. Intern Med J 2014;44(1):991–7.
83. Gunathilake R, Oldmeadow C, McEvoy M, et al. Mild hyponatremia is associated with impaired cognition and falls in community-dwelling older persons. J Am Geriatr Soc 2013;61:1838–9.
84. Gosch M, Joosten-Gstreen B, Heppner HJ, et al. Hyponatremia in geriatric inhospital patients. Gerontology 2012;58:430–40.
85. Brouns SH, Dortmans MK, Jonkers FS, et al. Hyponatraemia in elderly emergency department patients: a marker of frailty. Neth J Med 2014;72: 311–7.
86. Hoyle G, Chua M, Soiza R. Prevalence of hyponatremia in elderly patients. J Am Geriatr Soc 2006;54:1473–4.
87. Chua M, Hoyle GE, Soiza RL. Prognostic implications of hyponatremia in elderly hospitalized patients. Arch Gerontol Geriatr 2007;45:253–8.
88. Zenenberg RD, Carluccio AL, Merlin MA. Hyponatremia: evaluation and management. Hosp Pract (1995) 2010;38(1):89–96.
89. Jamal SA, Arampatzis S, Harrison SL, et al. Hyponatremia and fractures: findings from the Osteoporotic Fractures in Men study. J Bone Miner Res 2014. http://dx.doi.org/10.1002/jbmr. 2383.
90. Cervellin G, Mitaritonno M, Pedrazzoni M, et al. Prevalence of hyponatremia in femur neck fractures: a one-year survey in an urban emergency department. Adv Orthop 2014;2014:397059.

91. Gankham KF, Andres C, Sattar L, et al. Mild hyponatremia and risk of fracture in the ambulatory elderly. QJM 2008;101(7):583–8.
92. Sandhu HS, Gilles E, DeVita MV, et al. Hyponatremia associated with large-bone fracture in elderly patients. Int Urol Nephrol 2009;41(3):733–7.
93. Kinsella S, Moran S, Sullivan MO, et al. Hyponatremia independent of osteoporosis is associated with fracture occurrence. Clin J Am Soc Nephrol 2010;5(2):275–80.
94. Verbalis JG, Barsony J, Sigimura Y, et al. Hyponatremia-induced osteoporosis. J Bone Miner Res 2010;25(3):554–63.
95. Barsoney J, Xu Q, Sandberg T, et al. Chronic mild hyponatremia causes bone loss. Endocr Rev 2011;32:2–105.
96. Hoorn EJ, Liamis G, Zietse R, et al. Hyponatremia and bone: an emerging relationship. Nat Rev Endocrinol 2011;8(1):33–9.
97. Hagino T, Ochiai S, Watanabe Y, et al. Hyponatremia at admission is associated with in-hospital death in patients with hip fracture. Arch Orthop Trauma Surg 2013;133(4):507–11.
98. Tamma R, Sun L, Cuscito C, et al. Regulation of bone remodeling by vasopressin explains the bone loss in hyponatremia. Proc Natl Acad Sci U S A 2013;110(46):18644–9.
99. Buffington MA, Abreo K. Hyponatremia: a review. J Intensive Care Med 2015. [Epub ahead of print].
100. Nagler EV, Vanmassenhove J, van der Veer SN, et al. Diagnosis and treatment of hyponatremia: a systematic review of clinical practice guidelines and consensus statements. BMC Med 2014;12:1.
101. Cassagnol M, Shogbon AO, Saad M. The therapeutic use of vaptans for the treatment of dilutional hyponatremia. J Pharm Pract 2011;24(4):391–9.
102. Peri A. Clinical review: the use of vaptans in clinical endocrinology. J Clin Endocrinol Metab 2013;98(4):1321–32.

The Role of Nutrition and Physical Activity in Cholesterol and Aging

Sandra Maria Lima Ribeiro, PhD[a,*], Silmara dos Santos Luz, PhD[b], Rita de Cássia Aquino, PhD[c]

KEYWORDS

• Aging • Cholesterol • Lipoproteins • Atherogenesis • Alzheimer disease • Diet • Physical activity • Physical exercise

KEY POINTS

- Cholesterol is fundamental to biologic processes, and at the same time, alterations in cholesterol are associated with several diseases.
- During aging, diseases associated with cholesterol alterations (eg, atherosclerosis and Alzheimer disease) can assume special importance.
- Because of the variability in the aging process among individuals, pharmacologic interventions to reduce cholesterol can present negative outcomes.
- Healthy lifestyle interventions represent the best option for optimizing cholesterol levels, and should include a diet with an appropriate balance of macronutrients, with inclusion of natural foods and reduction in processed foods, and daily practice of at least 30 minutes of physical activity.

INTRODUCTION

Lipids, including cholesterol, are fundamental to health because they have structural and metabolic functions. The different lipids that compose the human body are the phospholipids, triacylglycerol (TAG), and cholesterol. Because of their insolubility in water, most lipids need to be carried by lipoproteins (LPs), which contain specific carriers, the apolipoproteins (APOs).[1,2] A description of recent findings in LPs and APOs is found in **Table 1**.

Disclosures: The authors declare they have no relevant financial relationship to disclose.
[a] Research Group of Nutrition, Physical Activity and Aging Processes, Department of Gerontology, University of São Paulo, Avenue Arlindo Bettio 1000, Ermelino Matarazzo, São Paulo, CEP 03828-000, Brazil; [b] Research Group of Nutrition, Physical Activity and Aging Processes, University of São Paulo, Avenue Arlindo Bettio 1000, Ermelino Matarazzo, São Paulo, CEP 03828-000, Brazil; [c] Nutrition Department, São Judas Tadeu University, Rua Taquari, 546-Mooca, São Paulo, CEP 03166-000, Brazil
* Corresponding author.
E-mail address: smlribeiro@usp.br

Clin Geriatr Med 31 (2015) 401–416
http://dx.doi.org/10.1016/j.cger.2015.04.010 geriatric.theclinics.com
0749-0690/15/$ – see front matter

Table 1
Description of lipoprotein subclasses, functions, and composition

Name	CM	VLDL	LDL	HDL	IDL	LP(a)
Subclasses[a]	Remnant CM (CM_{rem})	VLDL1 to VLDL3	LDL1 to LDL5	HDL2 and HDL3	—	LP(a)F, LP(a)B, LP(a)S1, LP(a)S2, LP(a)S3, and LP(a)S4[b]
Main functions	Transport of lipids (mainly TAG) from intestine to the tissues (CM) and from the circulation to the liver (CM_{rem})	Transport of lipids from liver to the tissues	This LP is result of VLDL after the action of LPL; it transports mainly cholesterol to tissues	Responsible for the reverse transport of cholesterol	This LP is result of VLDL after the action of LPL, and it is rapidly removed from the blood Studies have shown the atherogenic property of this LP	There is a body of evidence associating this lipoprotein to the progression of atherosclerotic plaque
Composition in proteins and lipids (%), and order of the different lipids	Protein = 1.5%–2.5%; lipids = 97%–99% (1-TAG; 2-PL; 3-CE; 4-FC)	Protein = 5%–10%; lipids = 90%–95% (1-TAG; 2-PL; 3-CE; 4-FC)	Protein = 20%–25%; lipids = 75%–80% (1-CE; 2-PL; 4-TAG; 5-FC)	Protein = 40%–45% (HDL2); 50%–55% (HDL3); lipids = 55% (HDL2); 50% (HDL3) (1-PL; 2-CE; 4-TAG; 5-FC)	Protein = 15%–20%; lipids = 80%–85% (1-TAG; 2-PL + CE; 3-FC)	Protein = 27%–30.9%; lipids = 77.6% (1-CE; 2-TAG; 3-TC; 4-PL)
Description of the main APOs	APOA-IV, APOB-48, APOC-II, APOC-III, APOE	APOB-100, APOC-I, APOC-II, APOC-III, APOE	APOB-100	APOA-I, APOA-II, APOA-IV, APOC-I, APOC-II, APOD, APOE Recent studies have identified proteins in HDL particles, such as MPO, and PON1 that complexes with APOA-I	APOB-100	APOB-100, APOA

Abbreviations: CE, cholesteryl esters; CM, chylomicron; FC, free cholesterol; HDL, high-density lipoprotein; IDL, intermediate-density lipoproteins; LDL, low-density lipoprotein; MPO, myeloperoxidase; PL, phospholipids; PON1, paraoxonase-1; VLDL, very-low-density lipoprotein.

[a] Different methods and techniques have been proposed to identify subclasses of the lipoproteins.

[b] The letters in the subclasses were attributed to the speed of mobility, compared to APOB100. B, similar mobility to APOB100; F, faster than APOB100; S, slower than APOB100.

Data from Refs.[3–5]

Cholesterol enters in the metabolism via de novo biosynthesis or from the diet. Cholesterol from the diet together with other digested lipids forms primary LPs, the chylomicrons, in enterocytes. The chylomicrons are secreted into the lymphatic system, reaching the systemic circulation, and transport lipids to the muscle and to adipose tissue, with an important action of the LP lipase (LPL). After the exchange of fatty acids, the remnant chylomicrons are captured by the liver and submitted to the action of hepatic LPL. Via the action of this enzyme, the liver uses a portion of the fatty acids for its own energy and the cholesterol is incorporated in its membranes; the second part of the cholesterol is used for bile synthesis; and the remaining lipids are re-esterified, forming very-low-density lipoprotein (VLDL).

The VLDLs transport TAG to the tissues and then are hydrolyzed by LPL in the circulation to form intermediate-density lipoprotein and low-density lipoprotein (LDL). These molecules are captured by hepatic or peripheral cells, via specific receptors (eg, LDL-R). Inside the cells, free cholesterol can be esterified by the action of acyl CoA cholesterol acyltransferase.[1,2] In those different cells, cholesterol participates in membrane synthesis, in steroid hormone production, in the synthesis of bile salts, and in vitamin D synthesis.[1,2]

High-density lipoprotein (HDL) is synthesized by the liver and the intestine, and transports cholesterol from tissues to the liver via the process of reverse transport of cholesterol (RCT). HDL also has other important functions, such as the removal of oxidized lipids from LDL, the inhibition of adhesion molecules and monocytes, and the stimulation of nitric oxide (NO) release.

To prevent cholesterol overload, different cells can generate oxidized derivatives of cholesterol, the oxysterols. These molecules decrease the half-life of cholesterol, and promote its degradation and excretion. Oxysterols are also important for stimulating RCT and bile acid synthesis.[6] **Fig. 1** summarizes the trajectory of cholesterol in the body, and **Box 1** describes some modifications in cholesterol metabolism with aging.

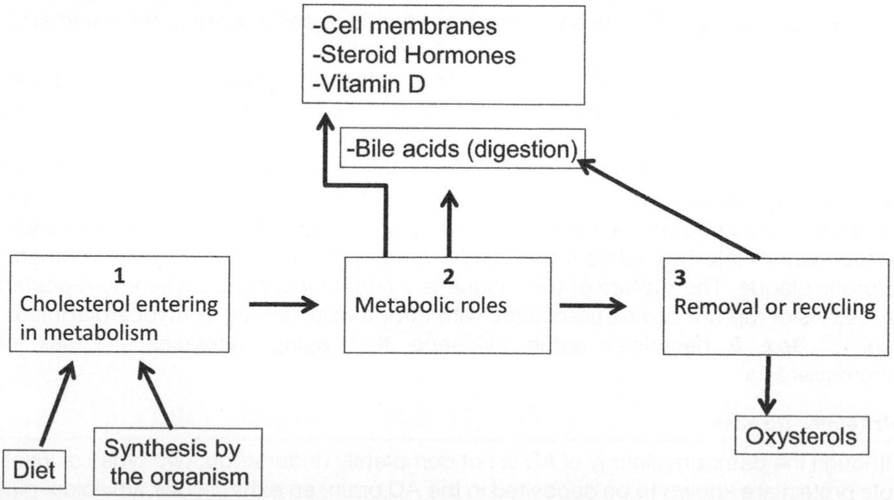

Fig. 1. Summary of the role of cholesterol in the human body.

Box 1
Aging and cholesterol

- With aging, there is an increase in the levels of atherogenic particles (mainly LDL); changes in HDL seem to be less significant.[7]
- There is also an increased production of oxysterols, which disturbs the NO-mediated mechanisms, leading to endothelial dysfunction and inflammation, inhibition of vascular relaxation, and increased blood pressure. Oxysterols also increase LDL oxidation.[6]
- Reduced levels of growth hormone, estrogens (menopause), thyroid hormones (common in women), and also elevated levels of cortisol contribute to altered expression of HMG-CoA reductase (a key enzyme in the cholesterol synthesis) and consequent LPs synthesis.[2]

Data from Refs.[2,6,7]

PATHOLOGIC CONDITIONS ASSOCIATED WITH CHOLESTEROL AND AGING

Aging is associated with several diseases, and cholesterol participates in some of the pathologic processes. This article discusses two pathologies: atherosclerosis and Alzheimer disease (AD).

Atherosclerosis

Atherosclerosis is an inflammatory process, occurring mainly in the intimal layer of medium- and high-caliber arteries, which develops progressively over the years, being the major cause of cardiovascular diseases (CVD; a group of disorders of the heart and blood vessels).[8]

Atherosclerosis starts with hypercholesterolemia, which is a result of accumulation of LDL in plasma, diminished hydrolysis of TAG, enhanced VLDL synthesis, or even a result of genetic defects.[2] Hypercholesterolemia is associated with endothelial dysfunction, leading to the increased permeability of the intima to LPs and their consequent retention, resulting in their subsequent oxidation. The oxidized LDL (LDLox) attracts leukocytes, such as monocytes and T lymphocytes, via interactions with their adhesion molecules. The monocytes differentiate into macrophages, which are responsible for the phagocytosis of LDLox. Once saturated with oxidized lipids, the macrophages are called foam cells, which are the main component of the atherosclerotic lesion.[9,10]

It has been proposed that LP(a) participates in the atherosclerotic lesion, together with LDL. LP(a) is more susceptible to oxidation than LDL, facilitating its capture by macrophages, and the formation of foam cells.[3]

With the progression of the atherosclerotic plaque, some inflammatory mediators stimulate the migration and proliferation of vascular smooth muscle cells and their secreted products from the arterial medium layer. These cells secrete cytokines and growth factors into the extracellular matrix, forming the fibrous cover of the atherosclerotic plaque. The rupture of this plaque is a constant process, whereby repeated processes of rupture can be associated with thrombosis, stroke, or myocardial infarction.[9,10] **Box 2** describes some evidence that aging increases the risk of atherosclerosis.

Alzheimer Disease

Although the pathophysiology of AD is not completely understood, two types of insoluble protein are known to be deposited in the AD brain: an extracellular amyloidal plaque (made basically from amyloid-β [Aβ] peptides, derived from the amyloidal

Box 2
Aging increases the risk of atherosclerosis

- Aging naturally favors the oxidation of lipoproteins, because of stress accumulation throughout life. As a consequence, the heart and vessels develop functional impairments, such as arterial stiffness, which makes recovery from the atherosclerotic plaques more difficult.[7]
- Molecular factors related to aged cells increase their vulnerability to atherosclerosis: changes in cell proliferative capacity; propensity to cell death; epigenetic modifications, such as histone acetylation and DNA mutilation; telomere shortening and dysfunction; increased formation from monocytes; and the activation and increased secretion of cytokines.[2]
- Increased oxysterol production and hormonal changes (see **Box 1**) favor the oxidation of LDL.
- Dyslipidemias are often secondary to other diseases typical of aging, such as hypothyroidism (mainly in women), diabetes or glucose intolerance, obesity, and hypertension.[11]

Data from Refs.[2,7,11]

precursor protein [APP]), and intracellular neurofibrillary tangles of hyperphosphorylated TAU protein.[12]

Raffai and Weisgraber[13] reviewed the evidence from epidemiologic, in vivo, and in vitro studies, and indicated cholesterol to be an important modulator of Aβ processing, contributing to AD. Next, we summarize the main hypothesis.

Brain cholesterol is locally synthesized, because the blood-brain barrier (BBB) prevents any contribution from plasma LPs. To cross the BBB (and then reach the liver to be metabolized and eliminated), brain cholesterol is converted to an oxysterol (24[S]-hydroxycholesterol). In AD, the concentration of 24(S)-hydroxycholesterol is higher than in individuals without AD. The increased flux of 24(S)-hydroxycholesterol is associated with neurodegeneration and neuronal death.[6]

The cleavage of APP occurs by two distinct pathways, with different enzymes. The first is the α-secretase. Cleavage by this enzyme originates two fragments: APPα and the carboxyl terminal. The other enzymes are β and γ secretases. These enzymes cleave two peptides, most with 40 amino acids (Aβ-40), and about 5% with 42 amino acids (Aβ-42). The latter is the most neurotoxic because it rapidly aggregates to form the insoluble amyloidal plaque. Although several proteases degrade Aβ-42, an enhanced production and/or an inefficient removal of Aβ-42 probably occurs in AD. Studies with animal models (mice expressing a mutant human APP) have shown that Aβ deposits, and reduced levels of APPsα, are proportional to enhanced plasma cholesterol. As such, it is hypothesized that hypercholesterolemia can alter APP processing by the α-secretase pathway, favoring the β and γ pathways.

It is possible, but not proved, that in hypercholesterolemia, LPs may leak into the brain through a damaged BBB, increasing neuronal cholesterol content and thereby affecting Aβ processing and cholesterol oxidation. One possible explanation for alterations in Aβ processing is that plasma membrane fluidity may enhance APP/α-secretase interactions, and in turn, rigid cholesterol-enriched membranes may reduce those interactions, favoring the action of γ-secretase.

The major APOs in the brain are APOE and APOA-I. APOE, derived from glial cells, provides lipids to neurons for membrane synthesis and repair, and is also important in processes of recovery from brain injury. APOE4 is less effective than its isoforms APOE3 or APOE2 in these processes, and the reasons for this are unknown. APOE4 is a risk factor for AD, accounting for 40% to 60% of the genetic variation of the disease; this isoform is probably more able to interact with Aβ, TAU, or the cytoskeleton.

Finally, epidemiologic data have shown a positive association between HDL level and cognition. In turn, various studies have found low levels of HDL in AD.[14]

PREVENTION OR TREATMENT OF HYPERCHOLESTEROLEMIA

Management of cholesterol levels in the elderly is important, and the oldest individuals deserve special attention. There are a high number of deaths caused by CVD in those older than 75 years. However, a review of observational studies shows reverse J-shaped or even U-shaped associations between total cholesterol (TC) and all-cause mortality, including CVD,[15,16] which means high mortality in the lowest TC.[16,17] These findings make the use of cholesterol-lowering treatments, such as statins, controversial for this population. In this context, prevention assumes a fundamental importance. A healthy diet, regular exercises, moderate use of alcohol, and nonsmoking are goals to be achieved, not only by the elderly, but by the population in general.

Cholesterol, Diet, and Aging

According to the World Health Organization (WHO)[18] a healthy diet is one "capable of being associated to a low prevalence of diet-related diseases in the population." Different studies have been conducted to identify the association between energy, nutrients, foods, or dietary patterns and chronic diseases. Some of these studies are described next.

Caloric Restriction

The restriction of calories in general has been the subject of several investigations. Despite controversies, studies with caloric restriction present interesting results, including cardiovascular benefits. Caloric restriction is capable of modulating the expression of sirtuins, especially sirtuin 1. The increase in sirtuin 1 improves vascular stiffness and attenuates the development of atherosclerosis, probably by activating endothelial NO synthase and promoting NO production.[19] Reasonable interventions of this type should evaluate the energy balance and discuss the possibilities of reducing caloric intake.

Dietary Fat

Most of the lipids from the diet are present in the form of TAG (1 glycerol + 3 fatty acids). Fatty acids can be classified according to the type of chemical bond and according to the chain size. Fatty acid nomenclature[20] is summarized in **Box 3**.

Fatty Acids

Saturated fatty acids

Effects The saturated fatty acids (SFA) are capable of increasing plasma cholesterol because of a reduction in hepatic LDL-R, inhibiting the plasma removal of this LP. However, stearic acid (18:0), which is present in cocoa (and dark chocolate), has a neutral or even cholesterol-lowering effect compared with other SFA.[21,22]

Food sources Sources include animal fats (meat, milk, and dairy products), certain plant oils (palm oils, coconut oils, and cocoa butter), and processed foods (cookies, cakes, doughnuts, and pies).

Additional comments Advices to reduce, or even to avoid red meat are very common in CVD prevention; however, such approaches are controversial. A recent investigation (EPIC cohort), including 448,568 participants in 10 European countries,

Box 3
Fatty acids in the human diet

- General fatty acid chemical classification is: saturated fatty acids (SFA), monounsaturated fatty acids (MUFA), polyunsaturated fatty acids (PUFA), and *trans*–fatty acids (TFA). However, some individual fatty acids within these groups have distinct biologic properties.
- SFAs in the diet are C14, C16, and C18 (long chain), with the exception of milk and coconut oil, where SFAs range from C4 to C18 (medium chain).
- The major MUFA in Western diets is oleic acid (C18:1n-9).
- The major PUFAs in the diet include linoleic acid (LA; C18:2n-6); a lower proportion of α-LA (ALA; C18:3n-3); and a variable proportion of long-chain PUFA, such as arachidonic acid (AA; 20:4 n-6), eicosapentaenoic acid (EPA; 20:5 n-3), and docosahexaenoic acid (DHA; 22:6 n-3).
- Therefore, we can enumerate:
  - n-3 fatty acids are ALA, EPA, and DHA
  - n-6 fatty acids are LA and AA
- The major TFAs in the diet are typically isomers of 18:1 *trans* derived from partially hydrogenated vegetable oils.

demonstrated that red meat intake was not significantly associated with CVD mortality, whereas processed meat was associated with 30% higher CVD.[23] In the "Asian prospective cohort studies,"[24] an inverse association was found between red meat intake and CVD mortality in men.

Milk and dairy products are also subject to intense discussions regarding CVD risk. Prospective observational studies and meta-analyses[25] showed no association and, in some cases, an inverse relationship between consumption of dairy products and the risk of different CVD. Two recent meta-analyses suggest that there is a significant inverse association between the intake of low-fat dairy products and the risk of type 2 diabetes.[26,27]

Regarding egg intake, two recent meta-analyses showed opposite results. The first, performed by Shin and colleagues,[28] did not show any relationship between eggs and CVD risk. The second study, conducted by Li and colleagues,[29] found positive associations between these parameters. Therefore, moderation could be the current keyword with regard to this issue.

Trans–fatty acids

Effects *Trans*–fatty acids are suggested to increase LDL and decrease HDL levels, to reduce the particle size of LDL cholesterol, to increase blood LP(a), and to increase inflammatory factors and adversely affect endothelial function. *Trans*–fatty acids are reported to have a higher atherogenic capacity than SFA.[21] An isomer of vaccenic acid (t11-c18:1) found in ruminant products is an exception because it has antiatherosclerotic properties.[30]

Food sources Sources include hydrogenated processed foods, and a lesser extent of animal products, such as meat and milk.

Cholesterol

Effects Cholesterol from diet can increase plasma cholesterol, but the response varies individually.

Food sources Sources include animal food in general: meats, eggs, and milk.

Additional comments The reduction in cholesterol in diet has long been argumentative. In the 1990s, after the American campaign to reduce cholesterol in the diet, controversial observations emerged. An association was suggested between a high level of depression, and even increased suicidal rates, with low cholesterol intake. Although not totally understood, it is possible that the depression rates occurring at that time resulted from a reduction in the total fat intake, especially polyunsaturated fatty acids (PUFA) and monounsaturated fatty acids (MUFA). It is known that low n-3, particularly docosahexaenoic acid, is responsible for the development of depression.[31]

Monounsaturated fatty acids

Effects MUFA is thought to decrease the oxidation of LDL, increase HDL, improve endothelial function and inflammation, and reduce prothrombotic environment.[32]

Food sources Sources include nuts, olive oil, some vegetable oils, and avocado.

Additional comments Virgin olive oil contains the MUFA oleic acid and some bioactive phytochemicals. Some epidemiologic studies have shown that the benefits of olive oil are caused by a combination of MUFA and these phytochemicals.[33]

In an interesting recent study, Oliveras-López and colleagues[34] evaluated the effects of daily consumption of extravirgin olive oil in healthy institutionalized elderly. Subjects (65–96 years) were divided into a control group who maintained their dietary habits and an olive group who consumed olive oil as the only added fat, plus a daily dose of 50 mL. They found a significant reduction in TC, LDL, and TAGs in the olive group, and a significant increase in HDL levels and improvements in antioxidant markers.

n-3 Polyunsaturated fatty acids

Effects n-3 PUFAs enhance LDL removal and reduce its hepatic production. They are also capable of reducing resting heart rate, blood pressure, and arrhythmia; they have an antiplatelet and antithrombotic effect, and improve endothelial function. n-3 PUFA has an anti-inflammatory effect, because it is capable of binding to peroxisome proliferator-activated receptor gamma, a ligand-activated transcription factor, which can modulate the nuclear factor-κB pathway and inhibit cytokine production.[35] However, caution is necessary in the intake of n-3 PUFAs, because they can increase potential of LDL to oxidation.[35]

Food sources Sources include oily fish (tuna, salmon, sardines, and herring), seafood, and some vegetable oils.

Additional comments The ORIGIN trial was a double-blind study that included older patients at a high risk for cardiovascular events and hyperglycemia. The participants received 900 mg of n-3 PUFAs or placebo daily. The study did not find any associations between n-3 PUFAs and major vascular events, death from any cause, or death from arrhythmia. The authors hypothesize that the studied population had a long history of exposure to CVD risk factors and diabetes, and the widespread use of preventive drugs, which could reduce the sensitivity to the supplement.[35] Therefore, the use of n-3 PUFA in older individuals deserves further investigation.

n-6 Polyunsaturated fatty acids

Effects n-6 PUFAs haves been shown to reduce LDL, to promote insulin sensitivity, and to reduce the risk of hypertension. However, there is some concern regarding its potential proinflammatory effects, because these can originate arachidonic acid, the initial molecule in inflammatory pathway. Farvid and colleagues[36] performed a systematic review and meta-analysis of prospective cohort studies to investigate the relationship between dietary linoleic acid (MUFA) intake and CVD risk. Thirteen eligible studies demonstrated dietary linoleic acid intake to be inversely associated with CVD risk in a dose-response manner.

Food sources Sources include vegetable oils (sunflower, safflower, soya, and corn) and nuts.

Additional comments Besides their n-6 PUFA content, nuts are also rich in MUFA, minerals and vitamins, and phenolic compounds and phytosterols. Intervention studies of walnuts showed them to decrease LDL and improve the TC/HDL-C ratio.[37]

Box 4 summarizes the effects of fatty acids on cholesterol.

Box 4
Summary of different fatty acids and their effects on cholesterol

- Dietary cholesterol has a modest effect on raising plasma cholesterol
- Dietary SFAs have a potent effect (via LDL) on raising plasma cholesterol
- PUFA (more potent) and MUFA have a cholesterol-lowering effect (via LDL)
- The cholesterol-raising effect of SFA is more potent than the cholesterol-lowering effect of PUFA
- SFA, MUFA, and PUFA have a modest HDL-raising effect
- *Trans*-fatty acids increase LDL more than SFA
- *Trans*-fatty acids do not elevate HDL

Adapted from Refs.[18,20,38]

Other Nutrients, Foods, and Dietary Patterns

Despite the importance of lipid (fatty acids) intake, the proportion of other macronutrients ingested and the presence of some micronutrients constitute a healthy diet. For instance, evidence shows inverse association of fruits and vegetables intake with several chronic diseases.[18] **Table 2** presents some recommendation for a healthy diet.[18,20,38]

Nutritional supplements

Because of the importance of diet in the prevention of chronic diseases, numerous functional foods and/or dietary supplements, or even food extracts, are now commercially available with allegations to improve health. It is important to highlight that the efficacy of most nutritional supplements has not been proved, and experimental results indicate that some substances differ when used as supplements, compared with when ingested in the food.[32,38] In fact, evidence implies that the total matrix of a food is more important than just its nutrient content, and a healthy diet should be recommended as fundamental for CVD prevention.[39] **Table 3** describes two examples of the studied supplements in the context of cardiovascular health.

Diet patterns

Studies show that the Mediterranean diet pattern is an excellent model of protection against chronic diseases, and most food guides for different countries are now based on this diet. One interesting recent version of the Mediterranean diet includes environmental and social aspects of feeding in their representation.[43] In particular, approaches for older people should include these aspects (**Fig. 2**).

Table 2
Some recommendation for a healthy diet

Nutrient/Food	Goal (% of the Energy Intake)	Comments
Total fat	15%–30%	
SFA	<10%	—
Total PUFA	6%–10%	—
n-6 PUFA	5%–8%	—
n-3 PUFA	1%–2%	—
TFA	<1%	—
MUFA	By difference	This is calculated as: total fat- (SFA + PUFA + TFA)
Total carbohydrates	55%–75%	The percentage of total energy available after taking into account that consumed as protein and fat
Free sugars	<10%	The term "free sugars" refers to all monosacharides and dissacharides added to foods by the manufacturer, cook, or consumer, plus sugar naturally present in honey, syrup, and fruit juices
Protein	10%–15%	More details at Joint WHO/FAO/UNU Expert consultation on Protein and Amino Acid Requirement in Human Nutrition, held in Geneva from April 9–16, 2002
Cholesterol	<300 mg/d	—
Sodium chloride (sodium)	<5 g/d	Salt should be iodized appropriately
Fruits and vegetables	≥400 g/d or 5 servings/d	Fruits and vegetables in general, beyond the concentration of antioxidants molecules, are rich in many phytochemicals, such as polyphenols, which together can be related to the prevention of many diseases
Total dietary fiber	From foods	High intake of dietary fiber (eg, nondigestible polysaccharides, naturally occurring resistant starch and oligosaccharides, and lignins in plants) is associated with a reduced cardiovascular risk
Nonstarch polysaccharides	From foods	Whole grain cereals, fruits, and vegetables are the preferred sources of nonstarch polysaccharides

Abbreviation: TFA, *trans*–fatty acid.

Data from WHO/FAO. Joint WHO/FAO Expert Consultation on Diet, Nutrition and the Prevention of Chronic Diseases (2002 Geneva, Switzerland): report of a Joint WHO/FAO Expert Consultation, Geneva, 28 January–1 February, 2002; and Badimon L, Vilahur G, Padro T. Nutraceuticals and atherosclerosis: human trials. Cardiovasc Ther 2010;28(4):202–15.

Table 3
Supplements supposed to be beneficial to cardiovascular health

Supplement	Comments
Antioxidants in general, including vitamin E	Supplementation with antioxidants (vitamins A, C, E, folic acid, β-carotene, selenium, zinc) is expected to have significant effect on atherosclerosis. In vitro studies with vitamin E show reduced uptake of LDLox by macrophages, among other effects. However, different meta-analyses have failed to demonstrate any significant benefit with antioxidant supplementation in humans.[38,40,41]
Resveratrol	Resveratrol is the most studied polyphenol in wine; red wine consumption has shown to prevent endothelial function, reducing endothelial cell apoptosis; to increase artery elasticity; and to modulate monocyte migration. In addition, animal experiments associate resveratrol with the activity of sirtuins.[7,42] However, studies conducted in humans supplementing resveratrol have not found consistent effects with regard to blood cholesterol lowering.

Data from Refs.[7,38,40–42]

Cholesterol, Physical Activity/Exercise and Aging

Physical inactivity is a primary cause of a myriad of chronic diseases, including CVD and dyslipidemias, and many studies and reviews have shown that physical activity and exercise at any intensity have important roles in the control of these diseases. **Table 4** presents some of the effects of different types of physical activity on risk factors to CVD.[45–48]

The American Heart Association[1] reinforces the importance of exercise for the prevention and treatment of CVD, and the WHO[18] recommends a minimum of 30 minutes

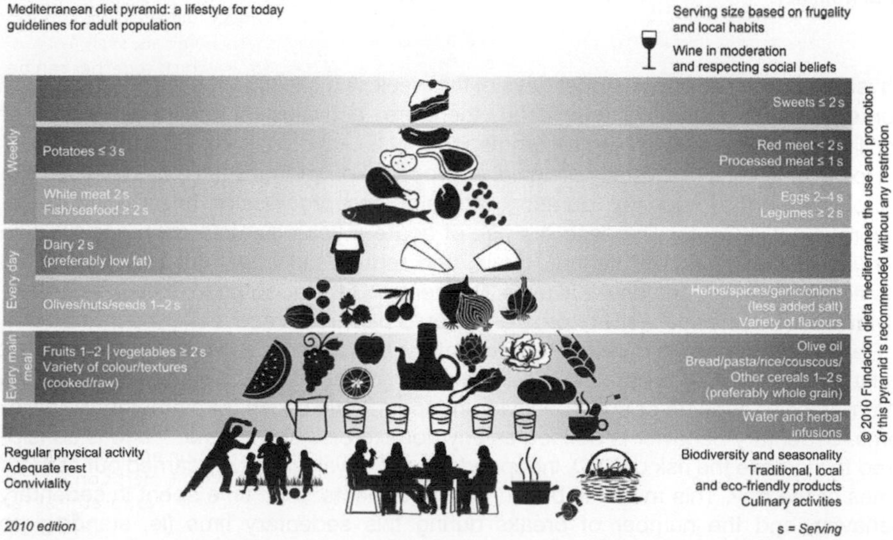

Fig. 2. Recent Mediterranean diet pyramid. Most food guides for different countries are based on Mediterranean diet pattern. (*Courtesy of* the Mediterranean Diet Foundation, Barcelona, Spain. Copyright © 2010 Fundación Dieta Mediterránea.)

Table 4
Effects of different types of physical activity on cholesterol management

Types of Physical Activity	Possible Effects	Intensity	Frequency and Duration
Aerobic activity	Aerobic physical activity may reduce LDL and non-HDL cholesterol, but has non consistent effect on HDL	Lower-intensity activities improve the energy metabolism of fatty acids	≥30 min/d most days of the week
		Moderate activities improve the energy metabolism of fatty acids, decrease oxidative stress, and decrease dyslipidemias	≥30 min/d most days of the week
		Vigorous activities decrease dyslipidemias, but is associated with decrease in spontaneous activity; risk of cardiac events in susceptible individuals, so supervision is recommended	≥30 min/d 3 d/wk
Resistance training	Resistance training may reduce LDL, TG, and non-HDL cholesterol, and has no consistent effect on HDL	—	3 d/wk
Sedentary behavior	Lack of physical activity affects almost every cell, organ, and system in the body causing dysfunctions and accelerated death		

Data from Refs.[2,10,18,44,45]

physical activity per day, on most days of the week. A higher volume and intensity may confer a better protective effect and, therefore, activities for the improvement of cardiorespiratory capacity are recommended.

However, given the diversity of aging, appropriate programs should be developed to adapt the mode, frequency, duration, intensity, and progression to each individual. Vigorous activities can increase the risk of acute myocardial infarction and sudden cardiac death in susceptible individuals, and require individual guidance, including medical evaluations and physical tests. Furthermore, the adaptation of each elderly individual to the physical activity program should be monitored.[1]

Recent studies have investigated sedentary behavior as a distinct standard that must be approached separately in relation to physical activity, because it is possible that particular aspects of such behavior independently cause cardiometabolic problems. Sedentary behavior is defined as any nonexercise sitting time,[44] and is considered to increase the risk of CVD, independently of physical activity carried out at other times of the day. This model is based on two aspects: total time spent in sedentary behavior, and the number of breaks during this sedentary time (ie, standing up from a resting or sitting position to a more active state, including standing). Both aspects are associated with cardiometabolic markers, independently of other lifestyle behaviors.[49]

Synthesis of Lifestyle Interventions to Manage Cholesterol and Aging

Box 5 summarizes the main goals for diet and physical activity to manage cholesterol in older persons.

Box 5
Summary of the main nonpharmacologic interventions to control cholesterol disturbances in older adults

- Diet should be varied and natural, including mainly fruits and vegetables, and avoiding processed foods. Culinary experiences to stimulate the ingestion of vegetables are beneficial to the elderly, especially individuals with reduced appetite.
- Having in mind the benefits and the criticisms of caloric restriction, the more reasonable practice is moderation in the intake of calories in general.
- According to evidence, a good strategy to reduce dyslipidemia is replacing sources of SFA by sources of MUFA and PUFA, which means a preference for food from vegetal sources, and preference for fish intake. However, the absolute restriction of any nutrient can result in nutritional disturbances; exclusion of specific foods, such as eggs, red meat, or milk, does not present evidence of benefit.
- Evidence does not show benefits of most of the commercial supplements; new products have to be discussed together with the physician and the dietitian.
- It is fundamental to be physically active; the minimum goal is to practice any type of physical activity, at least 30 minutes a day.

SUMMARY

Cholesterol is fundamental to several biochemical processes, and at the same time is related to several poor outcomes. Cholesterol management is fundamental for the control of CVD, especially during old age. This article discusses the main biologic processes that use cholesterol in the body, some pathologic events, and the major nonpharmacologic interventions to control cholesterol disturbances. In general, the goal should be a diet based on the Mediterranean-style diet; the choice of using nutritional supplements needs medical/dietitian evaluation. In addition, any type of physical activity seems to be beneficial; it is recommended at least 30 minutes a day, most days of the week.

REFERENCES

1. Eckel RH, Jakicic JM, Ard JD, et al. 2013 AHA/ACC guideline on lifestyle management to reduce cardiovascular risk. A report of the American College of Cardiology/American Heart Association Task Force on Practice Guidelines. J Am Coll Cardiol 2013;63(25 Pt B):2960–84.
2. de Cardiologia SB, Xavier HT, Izar MC, et al. V Diretriz Brasileira de dislipidemias e prevenção da aterosclerose. Arq Bras Cardiol 2013;101(1):1–20.
3. Maranhão RC, Carvalho PO, Strunz CC, et al. Lipoprotein (a): structure, pathophysiology and clinical implications. Arq Bras Cardiol 2014;103(1):76–84.
4. Diffenderfer MR, Schaefer EJ. The composition and metabolism of large and small LDL. Curr Opin Lipidol 2014;25(3):221–6.
5. Schaefer EJ, Anthanont P, Asztalos BF. High-density lipoprotein metabolism, composition, function, and deficiency. Curr Opin Lipidol 2014;25(3):194–9.
6. Zarrouk A, Vejux A, Mackrill J, et al. Involvement of oxysterols in age-related diseases and ageing processes. Ageing Res Rev 2014;18:148–62.

7. Cencioni C, Spallotta F, Mai A, et al. Sirtuin function in aging heart and vessels. J Mol Cell Cardiol 2015. [Epub ahead of print].
8. O'Flaherty M, Buchan I, Capewell S. Contributions of treatment and lifestyle to declining CVD mortality: why have CVD mortality rates declined so much since the 1960s? Heart 2013;99:159–62.
9. Hansson GK. Inflammation, atherosclerosis and coronary artery disease. N Engl J Med 2005;352(16):1685–95.
10. Libby P, Theroux P. Pathophysiology of coronary artery disease. Circulation 2005; 111(25):3481–8.
11. Wang JC, Bennett M. Aging and atherosclerosis: mechanisms, functional consequences, and potential therapeutics for cellular senescence. Circ Res 2012; 111(2):245–59.
12. Hardy J, Selkoe DJ. The amyloid hypothesis of Alzheimer's disease: progress and problems on the road to therapeutics. Science 2002;297:353–6.
13. Raffai RL, Weisgraber KH. Cholesterol: from heart attacks to Alzheimer's disease. J Lipid Res 2003;44(8):1423–30.
14. Hottman DA, Chernick D, Cheng S, et al. HDL and cognition in neurodegenerative disorders. Accumulating evidence indicates that the beneficial role of HDL extends to central nervous system. Neurobiol Dis 2014;72(Pt A):22–36.
15. Baigent C, Keech A, Kearney PM, et al. Efficacy and safety of cholesterol-lowering treatment: prospective meta-analysis of data from 90,056 participants in 14 randomised trials of statins. Lancet 2005;366:1267–78.
16. Petersen LK, Christensen K, Kragstrup J. Lipid-lowering treatment to the end? A review of observational studies and RCT on cholesterol and mortality in 80+ years old. Age Ageing 2010;39:674–80.
17. Casiglia E, Spolaore P, Ginocchio G, et al. Predictors of mortality in very old subjects aged 80 years or over. Eur J Epidemiol 1993;9:577–86.
18. WHO/FAO. Diet, nutrition and the prevention of chronic diseases: Report of the Joint WHO/FAO Expert Consultation. Geneva: World Health Organization; 2003 (WHO Technical Report Series 916).
19. Mellini P, Valente S, Mai A. Sirtuin modulators: an updated patent review (2012-2014). Expert Opin Ther Pat 2015;25(1):5–15.
20. FAO/WHO. Interim summary of conclusions and dietary recommendations on total fat & fatty acids from the Joint FAO/WHO Expert Consultation on Fats and Fatty Acids in Human Nutrition. Geneva (Switzerland): WHO HQ; 2008.
21. Hunter JE, Zhang J, Kris-Etherton PM. Cardiovascular disease risk of dietary stearic acid compared with trans, other saturated, and unsaturated fatty acids: a systematic review. Am J Clin Nutr 2010;91:46–63.
22. Mensink RP, Zock PL, Kester AD, et al. Effects of dietary fatty acids and carbohydrates on the ratio of serum total to HDL cholesterol and on serum lipids and apolipoproteins: a meta-analysis of 60 controlled trials. Am J Clin Nutr 2003;77: 1146–55.
23. Rohrmann S, Overvad K, Bueno-de-Mesquita H, et al. Meat consumption and mortality e results from the European Prospective Investigation into Cancer and Nutrition. BMC Med 2013;11:63.
24. Lee JE, McLerran DF, Rolland B, et al. Meat intake and cause-specific mortality: a pooled analysis of Asian prospective cohort studies. Am J Clin Nutr 2013;98: 1032–41.
25. Soedamah-Muthu SS, Verberne LD, Ding EL, et al. Dairy consumption and incidence of hypertension: a dose-response meta-analysis of prospective cohort studies. Hypertension 2012;60:1131–7.

26. Gao D, Ning N, Wang C, et al. Dairy products consumption and risk of type 2 diabetes: systematic review and dose-response meta-analysis. PLoS One 2013;8(9): e73965.
27. Aune D, Norat T, Romundstad P, et al. Dairy products and the risk of type 2 diabetes: a systematic review and dose-response meta-analysis of cohort studies. Am J Clin Nutr 2013;98:1066–83.
28. Shin JY, Xun P, Nakamura Y, et al. Egg consumption in relation to risk of cardiovascular disease and diabetes: a systematic review and meta-analysis. Am J Clin Nutr 2013;98:146–59.
29. Li Y, Zhou C, Zhou X, et al. Egg consumption and risk of cardiovascular diseases and diabetes: a meta-analysis. Atherosclerosis 2013;229:524–30.
30. Salter AM. Dietary fatty acids and cardiovascular disease. Animal 2013;7: 163–71.
31. Hibbeln JR, Salem N Jr. Dietary polyunsaturated fatty acids and depression: when cholesterol does not satisfy. Am J Clin Nutr 1995;62(1):1–9.
32. Garcia-Rios A, Delgado-Lista J, Alcala-Diaz JF, et al. Nutraceuticals and coronary heart disease. Curr Opin Cardiol 2013;28(4):475–82.
33. Ros E. Olive oil and CVD: accruing evidence of a protective effect. Br J Nutr 2012;108:1931–3.
34. Oliveras-López MJ, Molina JJ, Mir MV, et al. Extra virgin olive oil (EVOO) consumption and antioxidant status in healthy institutionalized elderly humans. Arch Gerontol Geriatr 2013;57(2):234–42.
35. Marchioli R, Levantesi G. n-3 PUFAs in cardiovascular disease. Int J Cardiol 2013;170:S33–8.
36. Farvid MS, Ding M, Pan A, et al. Dietary linoleic acid and risk of coronary heart disease: a systematic review and meta-analysis of prospective cohort studies. Circulation 2014;130(18):1568–78.
37. Ros E. Health benefits of nut consumption. Nutrients 2010;2:652–82.
38. Badimon L, Vilahur G, Padro T. Nutraceuticals and atherosclerosis: human trials. Cardiovasc Ther 2010;28(4):202–15.
39. Mente A, de Koning L, Shannon HS, et al. A systematic review of the evidence supporting a causal link between dietary factors and coronary heart disease. Arch Intern Med 2009;169:659–69.
40. Diaz MN, Frei B, Vita JA, et al. Antioxidants and atherosclerotic heart disease. N Engl J Med 1997;337:408–16.
41. The effect of vitamin E and beta carotene on the incidence of lung cancer and other cancers in male smokers. The alpha-tocopherol, beta carotene cancer prevention study group. N Engl J Med 1994;330:1029–35.
42. Williams RJ, Spencer JP. Flavonoids, cognition, and dementia: actions, mechanisms, and potential therapeutic utility for Alzheimer disease. Free Radic Biol Med 2012;52(1):35–45.
43. Bach-Faig A, Berry EM, Lairon D, et al. Mediterranean diet pyramid today. Science and cultural updates. Public Health Nutr 2011;12:2274–84.
44. Sedentary Behaviour Research Network. Letter to the editor: standardized use of the terms "sedentary" and "sedentary behaviours". Appl Physiol Nutr Metab 2012;37:540–2.
45. Wilcox S, Parra-Medina D, Thompson-Robinson M, et al. Nutrition and physical activity interventions to reduce cardiovascular disease risk in health care settings: a quantitative review with a focus on women. Nutr Rev 2001;59(7):197–215.
46. Ignarro LJ, Balestrieri ML, Napoli C. Nutrition, physical activity, and cardiovascular disease: an update. Cardiovasc Res 2007;73:326–40.

47. Booth FW, Roberts CK, Laye MJ. Lack of exercise is a major cause of chronic diseases. Compr Physiol 2012;2(2):1143–211.
48. Di Blasio A, Bucci I, Ripari P, et al. Lifestyle and high density lipoprotein cholesterol in postmenopause. Climacteric 2014;17(1):37–47.
49. Henson J, Yates T, Biddle SJ, et al. Associations of objectively measured sedentary behaviour and physical activity with markers of cardiometabolic health. Diabetologia 2013;56:1012–20.

Anorexia of Aging

Renuka Visvanathan, MBBS, FRACP, PhD

KEYWORDS

• Anorexia • Undernutrition • Sarcopenia • Older people

KEY POINTS

- Screening for appetite loss should occur.
- Those at risk should be assessed comprehensively.
- Medical, social, and other factors should be addressed.
- Exercise and good nutrition are important.

INTRODUCTION

The global population is aging and the proportion of older people is expected to double over the next century.[1] By 2050, 1 in every 6 people worldwide will be aged 65 years or older. Developing countries are aging more rapidly and in larger numbers than developed nations, and the segment of the population aged 60 years and older is expected to more than quadruple from 374 million to 1.6 billion between 2000 and 2050.

A major fear for older people everywhere is the loss of independence, and anything that can be done to prevent this loss would be highly valued. Undernutrition in older populations is a common health hazard that makes individuals more vulnerable to multiple health consequences that would threaten their independence. For example, impaired muscle function, decreased bone mass, immune dysfunction, anemia, reduced cognitive function, poor wound healing, delayed recovery from surgery, and increased mortality[2] can all result from poor diets, leading to hospitalization and residential care placement.[3,4] Residential care placement is an expensive and

Conflict of Interest: Professor R. Visvanathan is on the malnutrition in the elderly board, Nestle Australia, and has participated in international initiatives (ie, PROTAGE and MNA Initiative) made possible by educational grants by Nestle Inc. In the past, Professor R. Visvanathan has received educational and research grant funding from Organon Pty Ltd, Servier, Novartis, and Pfizer.

Aged & Extended Care Services, Level 8B, The Queen Elizabeth Hospital, Woodville Road, Woodville South, Adelaide, SA 5011, Australia
E-mail address: renuka.visvanathan@adelaide.edu.au

Clin Geriatr Med 31 (2015) 417–427
http://dx.doi.org/10.1016/j.cger.2015.04.012
geriatric.theclinics.com

distressing outcome for older people and their families, and it has long been clear that poor nutritional health is a major public health issue for all these reasons. The increase of the older population should therefore alert policy makers and health care providers to the imperatives of recognizing impaired nutritional status. Timely intervention to improve nutrition will benefit not just the individual and their family, but the whole community.

Anorexia is common in older people and is known to contribute to poor health owing to undesirable weight loss. This review focuses on describing the physiologic anorexia of aging in terms of prevalence, consequences, and pathophysiology. The review also offers practical management advice related to screening for anorexia in older people in the primary care setting.

WHAT IS THE ANOREXIA OF AGING?

The anorexia of aging refers to the physiologic reduction in appetite and food intake seen with advancing age.[5] This loss of appetite contributes to reduced nutrient intake that presages weight loss and undernutrition.[6] The average daily energy intake may decrease by up to 30% between the ages of 20 and 80 years.[6] For example, in the 1989 cross-sectional American National Health and Nutrition Examination Survey (NHANES III), a decline in energy intake of 1321 calories per day in men and 629 calories per day in women between the ages of 20 and 80 years was reported.[7] In older people, it is very important to note that many factors, often associated with aging, such as medication and illnesses, can also contribute to anorexia.[8]

Interestingly, it has been observed that anorexia in older people contributes to the reduction of intake of some but not all food groups.[9] Of particular concern for older people is the typical reduction in high-quality protein as a result of reduced consumption of meat, eggs, and fish.

It is wrong to think that this decrease in energy intake is an acceptable response to the natural decline in energy expenditure as people get older. Too often, the decrease in energy intake exceeds the decrease in energy expenditure, resulting in risky weight loss. With weight loss, there is often a concomitant loss of skeletal muscle mass (sarcopenia), which is of concern in older populations because healthy men and women in their seventh and eighth decades seem to be 20% to 40% weaker than their younger counterparts.[10]

Therefore, if left unchecked, the anorexia of aging may exacerbate the loss of muscle mass and strength, thus hastening the development of sarcopenia. And both the anorexia of aging and sarcopenia, when left unchecked, can result in the development of physical frailty,[8] a geriatric syndrome characterized by reduced homeostatic capacity to deal with stressors, such as acute illness, which develops as a result of an accumulation of deficits over a life span.[11]

PREVALENCE

The prevalence of the anorexia of aging as a physiologic condition separate from secondary causes of anorexia in older people is really not known, partly because there is little consensus as to the how best to make the diagnosis of anorexia. In 1 Italian study, researchers investigated the prevalence of anorexia in a random sample of older subjects aged 65 years and older living in the community (n = 217), in nursing homes (n = 213), and in rehabilitation and acute wards (n = 93).[9] In this study, anorexia was defined as a reduction in food intake, equal to or greater than 50% of the Italian recommended daily allowance over a 3-day period, and not attributable to secondary disorders of mastication, such as dysphagia or oral pain. The prevalence of anorexia was reported to be approximately 30% in the rehabilitation and acute wards and nursing homes. It was less common in the community, but approximately 11% of men and 3% of women were ingesting too few calories.

In another cross-sectional study of 1247 people aged 60 years and older in Mexico City, anorexia of aging was reported to be present in 30% of the study population, and associated with reduced mobility and disability.[12] Anorexia of aging in the study was considered to be an issue when a study participant reported eating less in the previous 12 months because of a loss of appetite.

SCREENING

The Simplified Nutritional Assessment Questionnaire (SNAQ) is a primary care, friendly tool consisting of only 4 questions relating to appetite, satiety, taste, and meal frequency, and is a suggested method of screening for anorexia and preventing future weight loss.[13] The questionnaire respondent is able to choose from 5 responses to each of the questions and the maximum score is 20. A risk score on the SNAQ is said to predict weight loss over a 6 months period with almost 82% sensitivity and 85% specificity for people aged 60 years and older.[13] Those scoring less than 15 out of 20 are said to be at risk of future weight loss.

PATHOPHYSIOLOGY

In comparison with younger people, healthy older people are less hungry, have early feelings of fullness, consume smaller and more monotonous meals, and eat fewer snacks between meals.[7,14] Some of the contributing factors to the changes in older persons' appetites are outlined in **Table 1**. These physiologic changes are said to be the root cause of the anorexia of aging.

Taste and Smell

Taste

The sense of taste is said to be commonly impaired with increasing age, especially after the age of 50 years.[5] In 1 study, more than 60% of subjects aged 65 to 80 years and more than 80% of subjects aged 80 years or older had major reductions in their sense of smell and this was in contrast with the 10% of subjects under 50 years of age affected by reductions in these senses.[15]

In general, there are 3 broad diagnostic categories to classify altered taste: *ageusia* (total loss of the sense of taste), *hypogeusia* (reduced ability to taste), and *dysgeusia* (distortion of the sense of taste).[16] Changes in the oral cavity that contribute to a reduced sense of taste include reduced mucosal thickness, increased dryness, reduced acini, increased fibrous adipose tissue in the salivary glands, and reduced density of the taste buds.[17] Diseases and medications further exacerbate the altered sense of taste in older age.

Smell

Food intake in older people, including the type of food eaten, is also affected by the decline in the sense of smell. The consequent, undesirable impact on food and beverage flavor results in a reduced interest in food while contributing to a change to a less varied and more monotonous diet.[18] Of concern, decreased olfactory function is said to be present in more than one-half of those aged between 65 and 80 years.[18]

The loss of sense of smell with advancing age is owing to multiple factors, including, but not limited to, changes in autonomic control of nasal engorgement, increased

Table 1
Some physiologic factors contributing to the anorexia of aging

Factors	Effects
Nonhormonal factors	
Diminished sense of smell and taste	Decreased oral intake
Reduced sensory specific satiety	More monotonous diet
Increased cytokine activity	Reduced food intake, catabolism, cachexia
Alteration in gastrointestinal function, delayed gastric emptying, Altered gastric distribution of food	Increased satiation and satiety
Hormonal factors	
Central	
Opioid: Decreased opioid activity, not proven in humans	Exogenous opioid increases food intake in adult humans
Neuropeptide Y: Possible decrease with aging, little evidence in humans	Not been administered in humans; increases food intake in animals
Galanin and orexin: its role is unclear	Not been administered in humans
Peripheral	
Cholecystokinin: satiating effects seem to increase with age	Exogenous administration reduces food intake in animal and humans
Ghrelin: increased in underweight and undernourished people	Exogenous administration stimulates food intake, gastric emptying and growth hormone release
Glucagonlike peptide-1 (*GLP-1*): effects of aging not fully understood	Administration in humans reduces food intake and increases feeling of fullness
Peptide YY: the effect of age on peptide YY is unclear	Administration reduces food intake and weight in human; not consistent finding
Leptin: leptin levels increase with aging but may be mostly explained by increase adiposity and reduced testosterone levels	Administration suppresses food intake and appetite

Data from Chapman IM. Endocrinology of anorexia of ageing. Best Pract Res Clin Endocrinol Metab 2004;18:437–52. MacIntosh C, Morley JE, Chapman IM. The anorexia of aging. Nutrition 2000;16:983–5.

presence of concomitant nasal disease, accumulated damage to the olfactory epithelium from lifelong environmental insults, decrease in protective enzymes in the olfactory mucosa, neurotransmitter and neuromodulator systems changes, and neuropathologic processes associated with neurodegenerative disorders, such as Alzheimer's dementia and Parkinson's disease.[18]

Cytokines

Cytokines may contribute to the development of anorexia. It is commonly asserted that aging itself is a form of stress resulting in increased cortisol and catecholamine levels, which in turn stimulate the release of inflammatory cytokines such as interleukin (IL)-6 and tumor necrosis factor-α.[5,19] Anorexia has been associated with cytokines, such as IL-1β, IL-6, and tumor necrosis factor-α.[20] In a study of healthy adults where there was no evidence of recent weight loss, Dent and colleagues[21] demonstrated that SNAQ scores were associated negatively with serum levels of proinflammatory IL-1β and associated positively with antiinflammatory cytokine IL-10. Therefore, changes in cytokine secretion may be contributing to anorexia well before any impact on body composition is noticed.

Altered Satiety and Satiation

Satiation is the process that leads to the termination of eating and may be accompanied by a feeling of satisfaction.[22] *Satiety*, on the other hand, is the feeling of fullness that persists after eating, potentially suppressing future energy intake until there is once again a feeling of hunger.[22] The satiety cascade describes how bodily functions influence satiation and satiety over time. Sensory and cognitive factors, including expectations about what is to be consumed—taste, smell, and texture—as well as past experience are initial influencers.[23] Once the nutrient reaches the stomach, gut distention signals the brain to initiate satiation. As nutrients travel into the intestines, gut hormones are released to promote satiation and satiety. Finally, in the postabsorptive stage, nutrients stimulate various sites in the body, including the brain, releasing signals that influence satiety.

With advancing age, the satiety cascade is altered. The shift to other food choices during a meal promoting the intake of a more varied, nutritionally balanced diet is related to sensory-specific satiety, the normal decline in pleasantness of the taste of a particular food after it has been consumed. However, older people, in contrast with younger people, have been shown to demonstrate impairment and therefore are less likely to naturally vary the nutrient content of meals; thus, they are at greater risk for developing undernutrition.[7]

Furthermore, cell loss within the mesenteric plexus of the esophagus, as well as a decline in the conduction velocity within visceral neurons, are associated with aging.[5] The ensuing reduction in sensory perception inhibits the positive stimuli for feeding and so, contributes to reduced food intake.

An increase in nitric oxide associated with aging is thought to play a role in the development of anorexia.[5] An impaired gastric accommodation response is seen because of altered fundic nitric oxide so that the relaxation of the proximal stomach is associated with rapid antral filling and earlier antral stretch, resulting in early satiation.[24,25] Decreased acid secretion and slower rates of gastric emptying have also been described in some, but not all, studies.[26]

Postprandial hunger seems to be related inversely to the rate of gastric emptying.[27] The advice to older people to eat smaller but more frequent meals is based on research findings showing that older people eating smaller meals exhibit the same gastric emptying rate as younger individuals.[5] Gut transit time and postprandial motility seem not to be affected in healthy older people. However, increases in frequency and amplitude of isolated pressure waves in older people compared with younger people have been noted previously and is thought to possibly contribute to a reduced feeling of satiation following a meal.[28]

Neuroendocrine Mechanisms

Appetite and food intake are also dependent on the neuroendocrine axis, which includes the *central hormones*, represented by opioids, neuropeptide Y, galanin, and the orexins; and *peripheral hormones*, including gut peptides and adipose tissue secreted hormones, represented by cholecystokinin (CCK), ghrelin, glucagonlike peptide-1 (GLP-1), peptide YY (PYY), leptin, adiponectin, resistin, insulin, glucagon, amylin, corticotrophin-releasing factor, and serotonin. A brief discussion of these mechanisms is offered here, and a more detailed review on this topic is available elsewhere.[5]

Central hormones

Opioids There may be a reduced opioid feeding drive associated with aging.[24] Lower plasma and cerebrospinal fluid ß-endorphin concentrations have been noted in older patients with idiopathic, senile anorexia compared with normal weight, aged-matched controls.[29]

Neuropeptide Y Neuropeptide Y (NPY) is synthesized in the brain and peripheral nervous system and strongly stimulates food intake. Plasma and cerebrospinal fluid levels of NPY are increased in elderly people with idiopathic anorexia.[29] It is for this reason that NPY has been implicated in the development of the anorexia of aging.

Galanin Galanin, a peptide hormone located in the peripheral nervous system and brain, stimulates food intake. Reduced sensitivity to galanin is thought to contribute to the anorexia of aging.[30]

Orexins (hypocretins) Involved with sleep and eating, orexin A and B (hypocretin-1 and –2) are neuropeptides synthesized in the hypothalamus. The effect of age on brain and receptor levels and the sensitivity to orexin is not known, but plasma orexin concentrations increase with age in healthy adults.[31] Orexin has also been shown to stimulate robust food intake in rats.[32]

Peripheral hormones, including gut peptides and adipose tissue secreted hormones

Gut peptides

Cholecystokinin Released from the lumen of the intestine in response to nutrients in the gut, particularly fat and protein, CCK is present in the hypothalamus, cortex, and midbrain.[5] Smaller meal sizes are related to higher levels of CCK, which is not surprising, given the observation that the production of plasma CCK concentrations within a certain physiologic range results in the suppression of food intake. The converse is observed with the administration of CCK antagonists.[33]

CCK coordinates the release of digestive enzymes while slowing gastric emptying. With advancing age, the increased signaling of CCK contributes to the suppression of food intake and ultimately weight loss.[34] Elderly people with idiopathic anorexia have significantly higher plasma levels and not significantly higher cerebrospinal fluid levels of CCK compared with healthy, age-matched controls.[29]

The administration of CCK suppresses food intake twice as much in healthy older adults than in healthy young adults.[34] There may also be age-related resistance to the appetite suppressing effects of CCK, given that older people are more sensitive to the effects of increased levels of CCK than younger people, and also have higher fasting concentrations of CCK.[34]

Ghrelin Present in the hypothalamus, ghrelin is produced predominantly in the stomach and stimulates growth hormone release. Peripheral infusion of ghrelin in humans is known to stimulate appetite.[35] Mild adverse effects are common following ghrelin administration and affects 20% of people studied. These effects include flushing and gastric rumbles. In healthy adults, plasma ghrelin levels have been shown to be correlated inversely with skeletal muscle mass but not with age or energy intake.[36] However, in some other studies, plasma ghrelin levels have been shown to negatively correlate, albeit weakly, with advancing age.[37]

Glucagonlike peptide-1 GLP-1, which is released by the lining of the intestine in response to nutrient ingestion, such as carbohydrates, slows gastric emptying, and stimulates insulin together with gastric inhibitory peptide secretion.[5] Administration of GLP-1 to humans reduces food intake and increases feelings of fullness.[38] The effects of aging on the satiating effects of GLP-1 and the effects of aging on plasma GLP-1 concentrations are not conclusively understood.[39]

Peptide YY PYY, which is present also in the brain, is a peptide hormone released from the bowel in response to the detection of fat and carbohydrate in the small intestine. Intravenous infusion of PYY that produces postprandial blood levels has been shown to reduce short-term food intake in normal weight and obese adults (<50 years) by approximately 30%, but the results of this 1 study have not been reproduced.[40] It is, therefore, unclear whether PYY truly contributes to the development of the anorexia of aging.[5]

Adipose tissue released hormones

Leptin Leptin is an anorexigenic hormone released by the adipose tissue, and its circulating amount is directly related to the size of fat stores. With advancing age, there is increased adiposity; therefore, it is no surprise that plasma leptin concentrations in humans increase as people become older.[41] Levels of leptin may also increase as a result of a decline in serum testosterone levels in men. It has been shown that testosterone therapy reduces, and inhibition of testosterone secretion increases, leptin levels.[42] Interestingly, and possibly related to leptin resistance, leptin administration in obese people results only in minor weight loss.[5]

Adiponectin Adiponectin, secreted from adipose tissue, is involved in glucose regulation and fatty acid oxidation. Adiponectin levels have been shown to correlate positively with age but negatively with the body mass index.[43] Its role in the development of the anorexia of aging is unclear.

Resistin Expressed in white adipose tissue, resistin reduces energy intake by affecting NPY neurons and suppresses insulin-simulated glucose uptake in fat tissue.[44] Its role in the anorexia of aging has not been investigated.

Pancreatic hormones

Insulin Insulin is a satiety signal that reduces food intake by acting on the arcuate nucleus of the lateral hypothalamus. Increases in fasting and postprandial circulating insulin concentrations are noted with aging.[45] In part, insulin resistance as a result of increased adiposity is the major contributing factor to the age-associated increase in insulin concentrations. Not only have some studies reported increased basal insulin levels in the older population, but a greater increase in blood glucose and insulin levels is seen after intraduodenal glucose infusions in the elderly compared with the young.[26,46]

Glucagon and amylin Glucagon is postulated to reduce meal size by increasing glucose oxidation for energy in rats but, to date, there has been no research related to glucagon administration.[26,47] Amylin, produced by the beta islet cells in the pancreas, has been investigated as an antiobesity agent, reduces gastric emptying and also energy intake through a direct effect on the hypothalamus.[48] However, it is unclear whether age-related changes to amylin levels or effects occur, or if amylin plays a role in the development of the anorexia of aging.[26]

MANAGING ANOREXIA TO ACHIEVE HEALTHY AGING

There is limited evidence to support the use of any form of pharmacologic treatment routinely to treat anorexia in older people. Instead, the use of a comprehensive approach when managing older people will most likely lead to desirable health care outcomes, which promote independence and quality of life.

It is important to screen for appetite loss (eg, using the SNAQ) whenever the opportunity arises during interaction with older people in a health care setting. Early intervention may prevent future weight loss and the commonly associated health deterioration over time. As already alluded to, anorexia in older age can be owing to secondary causes, including medical reasons. In a study of 1904 nursing home residents in Italy, reversible factors such as depression, pharmacologic therapies, and chewing problems were associated strongly with anorexia, which was defined as low food intake or the presence of low appetite.[49] Anorexia in the study was associated independently with increased mortality.

It is therefore vital, where risk is noted, to undertake a comprehensive history and physical examination, identifying and addressing potentially remediable factors. Medical, emotional, social, and environmental factors should be investigated. Failure to address contributing factors will result in failure to prevent deterioration or bring about improvement.

Among the issues that are likely to be detected during a thorough examination is the loss of smell or taste. The reduction in these senses is difficult to manage. One recent study found that flavor intensification did not alter sensory-specific satiety.[50] However, other studies have found that the addition of flavor enhancers, such as sauce to food or glutamate, may be of benefit in terms of nutritional intake and therefore such strategies are worth trying.[51–53]

Another important strategy is to encourage activities that promote wellness across the lifespan. This strategy should be incorporated as part of public health campaigns that aim to maintain health into older age, allowing older people to achieve healthy aging. Encouraging older people to build up their muscle reserves will help to ensure greater resilience if they are challenged with illness.

Aerobic as well as resistance exercise positively impacts on muscle mass and strength.[54] It is also well-documented that it is never too late to start. Older people can benefit from exercise even in their eighth or ninth decade of life.[54] Group exercise classes may contribute to socialization, and exercise is likely to have a positive impact on nutritional intake and mood.[55]

It is currently recommended that healthy older people should consume at least 1.2 g/kg body weight per day. Also, it is further recommended that up to 25 g of protein be consumed with each of the 3 main meals.[54] Where possible, older people should aim to meet these requirements through natural food products. They should also ensure that caloric requirements, as well as other nutrient requirements (eg, fruits, fiber), are also met.

If anorexia of aging has been detected, however, meeting the necessary protein requirements may be a challenge for older and frail individuals. Even if they understand what is happening to their appetite and weight, it is extremely difficult to eat when they are not hungry or particularly interested in food. For this at-risk group, the use of nutritional supplements with a high protein content, might be an important strategy to be considered. High-protein drinks may be required at a main meal for particularly susceptible individuals.

However, some researchers have expressed concerns that the administration of nutritional supplements at meal time may actually compromise food intake during the meal, thus reducing overall caloric intake. Furthermore, compliance with milk-based supplements can be hampered by gastrointestinal side effects, which can sometimes be addressed by splitting the drink into smaller quantities or using a lactose-free supplement. Along with small quantities of nutritional supplements, snacks between meals have been suggested to achieve total caloric intake.

The beneficial effects of nutritional supplements on preserving physical function are not conclusive, however, and further research is required to investigate this, because currently these supplements are not subsidized and can be very costly, further limiting their use.

SUMMARY

Anorexia in older people is common and can contribute to weight loss, sarcopenia, and poor health outcomes. Not only are there gut and neuroendocrine changes that contribute to the development of the anorexia of aging, but there are many other factors that should be addressed if the adverse consequences arising from the anorexia of aging are to be prevented. Exercise and adequate protein intake are important public health measures that should be strategically and enthusiastically encouraged, because they will better provide older people with reserves to withstand future health stressors. Currently, there is no convincing evidence to support pharmacologic interventions to prevent or treat the anorexia of aging.

REFERENCES

1. World Population Ageing 1950–2020. II. Magnitude and speed of population ageing. In: Department of Economic and Social Affairs of the United Nations PD, editor. New York: 2001. Available at: http://www.un.org/esa/population/publications/worldageing19502050/pdf/80chapterii.pdf. Accessed April 07, 2015.
2. Visvanathan R. Under-nutrition in older people: a serious and growing global problem! J Postgrad Med 2003;49:352–60.
3. Visvanathan R, Macintosh C, Callary M, et al. The nutritional status of 250 older Australian recipients of domiciliary care services and its association with outcomes at 12 months. J Am Geriatr Soc 2003;51:1007–11.
4. Visvanathan R, Penhall R, Chapman I. Nutritional screening of older people in a sub-acute care facility in Australia and its relation to discharge outcomes. Age Ageing 2004;33:260–5.
5. Chapman IM. The anorexia of aging. Clin Geriatr Med 2007;23:735–56, v.
6. Omran ML, Morley JE. Assessment of protein energy malnutrition in older persons, Part II: laboratory evaluation. Nutrition 2000;16:131–40.
7. Rolls BJ, McDermott TM. Effects of age on sensory-specific satiety. Am J Clin Nutr 1991;54:988–96.
8. Martone AM, Onder G, Vetrano DL, et al. Anorexia of aging: a modifiable risk factor for frailty. Nutrients 2013;5:4126–33.
9. Donini LM, Poggiogalle E, Piredda M, et al. Anorexia and eating patterns in the elderly. PLoS One 2013;8:e63539.
10. Doherty TJ. Invited review: aging and sarcopenia. J Appl Physiol 2003;95:1717–27.
11. Clegg A, Young J, Iliffe S, et al. Frailty in elderly people. Lancet 2013;381:752–62.
12. Vazquez-Valdez OE, Aguilar-Navarro S, Avila-Funes JA. Association between anorexia of aging and disability in older community-dwelling Mexicans. J Am Geriatr Soc 2010;58:2044–6.
13. Wilson MM, Thomas DR, Rubenstein LZ, et al. Appetite assessment: simple appetite questionnaire predicts weight loss in community-dwelling adults and nursing home residents. Am J Clin Nutr 2005;82:1074–81.
14. Visvanathan R, Chapman IM. Undernutrition and anorexia in the older person. Gastroenterol Clin North Am 2009;38:393–409.
15. Doty RL, Shaman P, Applebaum SL, et al. Smell identification ability: changes with age. Science 1984;226:1441–3.

16. Kettaneh A, Paries J, Stirnemann J, et al. Clinical and biological features associated with taste loss in internal medicine patients. A cross-sectional study of 100 cases. Appetite 2005;44:163–9.
17. Imoscopi A, Inelmen EM, Sergi G, et al. Taste loss in the elderly: epidemiology, causes and consequences. Aging Clin Exp Res 2012;24:570–9.
18. Doty RL, Kamath V. The influences of age on olfaction: a review. Front Psychol 2014;5:20.
19. Yeh SS, Schuster MW. Geriatric cachexia: the role of cytokines. Am J Clin Nutr 1999;70:183–97.
20. Morley JE, Baumgartner RN. Cytokine-related aging process. J Gerontol A Biol Sci Med Sci 2004;59:M924–9.
21. Dent E, Yu S, Visvanathan R, et al. Inflammatory cytokines and appetite in healthy people. J Aging Research Clin Pract 2012;1(1):40–3.
22. Benelam B. Satiety and the anorexia of ageing. Br J Community Nurs 2009;14: 332–5.
23. Blundell JE, Rogers PJ, Hill AJ. Evaluating the satiating power of foods: implications for acceptance and consumption. In: Solms J, Booth DA, Pangbourne RM, et al, editors. Food acceptance and nutrition. London: Academic Press; 1987. p. 205–19.
24. Morley JE. Anorexia of aging: physiologic and pathologic. Am J Clin Nutr 1997; 66:760–73.
25. Morley JE. Decreased food intake with aging. J Gerontol A Biol Sci Med Sci 2001; 56(Spec No 2):81–8.
26. Atalayer D, Astbury NM. Anorexia of aging and gut hormones. Aging Dis 2013;4: 264–75.
27. Clarkston WK, Pantano MM, Morley JE, et al. Evidence for the anorexia of aging: gastrointestinal transit and hunger in healthy elderly vs young adults. Am J Physiol 1997;272:R243–8.
28. Cook CG, Andrews JM, Jones KL, et al. Effects of small intestinal nutrient infusion on appetite and pyloric motility are modified by age. Am J Physiol 1997;273:R755–61.
29. Martinez M, Hernanz A, Gomez-Cerezo J, et al. Alterations in plasma and cerebrospinal fluid levels of neuropeptides in idiopathic senile anorexia. Regul Pept 1993;49:109–17.
30. Baranowska B, Radzikowska M, Wasilewska-Dziubinska E, et al. Relationship among leptin, neuropeptide Y, and galanin in young women and in postmenopausal women. Menopause 2000;7:149–55.
31. Matsumura T, Nakayama M, Nomura A, et al. Age-related changes in plasma orexin-A concentrations. Exp Gerontol 2002;37:1127–30.
32. Choi DL, Davis JF, Fitzgerald ME, et al. The role of orexin-A in food motivation, reward-based feeding behavior and food-induced neuronal activation in rats. Neuroscience 2010;167:11–20.
33. Beglinger C, Degen L, Matzinger D, et al. Loxiglumide, a CCK-A receptor antagonist, stimulates calorie intake and hunger feelings in humans. Am J Physiol Regul Integr Comp Physiol 2001;280:R1149–54.
34. MacIntosh CG, Morley JE, Wishart J, et al. Effect of exogenous cholecystokinin (CCK)-8 on food intake and plasma CCK, leptin, and insulin concentrations in older and young adults: evidence for increased CCK activity as a cause of the anorexia of aging. J Clin Endocrinol Metab 2001;86:5830–7.
35. Garin MC, Burns CM, Kaul S, et al. Clinical review: the human experience with ghrelin administration. J Clin Endocrinol Metab 2013;98:1826–37.
36. Tai K, Visvanathan R, Hammond AJ, et al. Fasting ghrelin is related to skeletal muscle mass in healthy adults. Eur J Nutr 2009;48:176–83.

37. Serra-Prat M, Fernandez X, Burdoy E, et al. The role of ghrelin in the energy homeostasis of elderly people: a population-based study. J Endocrinol Invest 2007; 30:484–90.
38. Flint A, Raben A, Astrup A, et al. Glucagon-like peptide 1 promotes satiety and suppresses energy intake in humans. J Clin Invest 1998;101:515–20.
39. MacIntosh CG, Andrews JM, Jones KL, et al. Effects of age on concentrations of plasma cholecystokinin, glucagon-like peptide 1, and peptide YY and their relation to appetite and pyloric motility. Am J Clin Nutr 1999;69:999–1006.
40. Batterham RL, Cohen MA, Ellis SM, et al. Inhibition of food intake in obese subjects by peptide YY3-36. N Engl J Med 2003;349:941–8.
41. Baumgartner RN, Waters DL, Morley JE, et al. Age-related changes in sex hormones affect the sex difference in serum leptin independently of changes in body fat. Metabolism 1999;48:378–84.
42. Hislop MS, Ratanjee BD, Soule SG, et al. Effects of anabolic-androgenic steroid use or gonadal testosterone suppression on serum leptin concentration in men. Eur J Endocrinol 1999;141:40–6.
43. Cnop M, Havel PJ, Utzschneider KM, et al. Relationship of adiponectin to body fat distribution, insulin sensitivity and plasma lipoproteins: evidence for independent roles of age and sex. Diabetologia 2003;46:459–69.
44. Steppan CM, Lazar MA. The current biology of resistin. J Intern Med 2004;255: 439–47.
45. Fraze E, Chiou YA, Chen YD, et al. Age-related changes in postprandial plasma glucose, insulin, and free fatty acid concentrations in nondiabetic individuals. J Am Geriatr Soc 1987;35:224–8.
46. Sturm K, MacIntosh CG, Parker BA, et al. Appetite, food intake, and plasma concentrations of cholecystokinin, ghrelin, and other gastrointestinal hormones in undernourished older women and well-nourished young and older women. J Clin Endocrinol Metab 2003;88:3747–55.
47. Geary N, Le Sauter J, Noh U. Glucagon acts in the liver to control spontaneous meal size in rats. Am J Physiol 1993;264:R116–22.
48. Brunetti L, Recinella L, Orlando G, et al. Effects of ghrelin and amylin on dopamine, norepinephrine and serotonin release in the hypothalamus. Eur J Pharmacol 2002;454:189–92.
49. Landi F, Lattanzio F, Dell'Aquila G, et al. Prevalence and potentially reversible factors associated with anorexia among older nursing home residents: results from the ULISSE project. J Am Med Dir Assoc 2013;14:119–24.
50. Havermans RC, Geschwind N, Filla S, et al. Sensory-specific satiety is unaffected by manipulations of flavour intensity. Physiol Behav 2009;97:327–33.
51. Appleton KM. Increases in energy, protein and fat intake following the addition of sauce to an older person's meal. Appetite 2009;52:161–5.
52. Prescott J. Effects of added glutamate on liking for novel food flavors. Appetite 2004;42:143–50.
53. Schiffman SS, Warwick ZS. Effect of flavor enhancement of foods for the elderly on nutritional status: food intake, biochemical indices, and anthropometric measures. Physiol Behav 1993;53:395–402.
54. Bauer J, Biolo G, Cederholm T, et al. Evidence-based recommendations for optimal dietary protein intake in older people: a position paper from the PROT-AGE Study Group. J Am Med Dir Assoc 2013;14:542–59.
55. Tse MM, Tang SK, Wan VT, et al. The effectiveness of physical exercise training in pain, mobility, and psychological well-being of older persons living in nursing homes. Pain Manag Nurs 2013;15:778–88.

Screening for Malnutrition in Older People

Sophie Guyonnet, PhD[a,b,c,*], Yves Rolland, MD, PhD[a,b,c]

KEYWORDS

• Malnutrition • Nutrition screening • Elderly

KEY POINTS

- The cumulative effect of the interaction between nutrition and changes seen in aging is *progressive* malnutrition, which often goes undiagnosed.
- Malnutrition poses a huge economic cost to society. Early detection is important because the malnourished elderly are more likely to require health and social services and have more hospitalizations and higher morbidity and mortality rates.
- There is no international consensus on a single best tool to screen malnutrition. The use of different tools in different studies hinders the comparison between studies.
- Older adults in long term-care facilities are at greatest nutritional risk, with malnutrition more likely among older residents and/or those who require a higher level of care.
- Earlier identification and appropriate nutrition support may help to reverse or halt the malnutrition trajectory and the negative outcomes associated with poor nutritional status.
- A nutrition screening process is recommended to help detect people with protein-energy malnutrition or at malnutrition risk. Any weight loss is a warning sign of malnutrition in elderly.

Malnutrition risk increases with age and level of care. Despite significant medical advances, malnutrition remains a significant and highly prevalent public health problem of developed countries. Malnutrition significantly increases morbidity and mortality and compromises the outcomes of other underlying conditions and diseases. Estimates of the prevalence vary, as methods for detection are not standardized. Early detection may lead to earlier intervention and improved outcomes and better quality of life. Thus, nutrition screening leading to the identification of etiologic factors is a necessary step. A single cause may rarely explain malnutrition in older adults, so it requires a systematic and multidisciplinary approach to identify all various causes usually involved. Several educational tools may facilitate the identification of factors

[a] Gérontopôle, Toulouse University Hospital, 170 avenue de Casselardit, TSA 40031, 31059 Toulouse cedex 9, France; [b] INSERM UMR 1027, 37 allées Jules Guesde, 31000 Toulouse cedex, France; [c] Université de Toulouse III Paul Sabatier University, 133 route de Narbonne, 31062 Toulouse cedex, France

* Corresponding author. Gérontopôle, Toulouse University Hospital, 170 avenue de Casselardit, TSA 40031, 31059 Toulouse cedex 9, France.

E-mail address: guyonnet.s@chu-toulouse.fr

Clin Geriatr Med 31 (2015) 429–437
http://dx.doi.org/10.1016/j.cger.2015.04.009 geriatric.theclinics.com
0749-0690/15/$ – see front matter

associated with malnutrition. Academic societies proposed different checklists to guide the diagnostic approach or interventions. Several valid malnutrition screening tools are available to identify nutritional risk, including:

- Mini Nutritional Assessment (MNA)[1–3]
- Malnutrition Screening Tool (MST)[4]
- Malnutrition University Screening Tool (MUST)[5]
- Nutritional Risk Screening 2002 (NRS 2002)[6]
- Subjective Global Assessment (SGA)[7]
- Simplified Nutritional Assessment Questionnaire (SNAQ)[8]

For elderly with protein-energy malnutrition (PEM) or at nutritional risk, evidence supports that oral nutritional supplements and dietary counseling can increase dietary intake and improve quality of life.

This article examines nutritional screening and assessment tools designated for older adults. The authors first summarize the current literature regarding the prevalence, cause, and consequences of malnutrition. Within this review, the term *malnutrition* refers primarily to PEM. PEM is caused by an imbalance between intake in the body's requirements. This imbalance causes tissue loss, in particular of muscle tissue, with harmful functional consequences.

The main educational objectives of this article are to address the following questions:

1. Who are the elderly at risk of malnutrition and/or what are the risk factors?
2. What tools may be used to detect and diagnose malnutrition in the elderly?

PREVALENCE OF MALNUTRITION IN ELDERLY

The older population remains heterogeneous and is currently categorized into *disabled* (if needing assistance to perform basic activities of daily living), *frail*, and *robust*. Frailty is a multidimensional geriatric syndrome characterized by increased vulnerability to stressors as a result of reduced capacity of different physiologic systems.[9] Several operational definitions of frailty are currently available in the literature. However, the most commonly used criteria are those proposed by Fried and colleagues,[9] defining the so-called frailty phenotype. This phenotype is determined by the presence of at least 3 of 5 signs/symptoms, including poor muscle strength, slow gait speed, unintentional weight loss, exhaustion, and sedentary behavior. A prefrail stage, in which one or 2 criteria are present, identifies a subset at high risk of progressing to frailty. Estimates of the prevalence of malnutrition vary, as methods for detection are not standardized. Additionally, it is known that the prevalence of malnutrition depends on the setting and increases as the level of care increases. Multicenter studies that have evaluated malnutrition prevalence in the acute care setting report that 23% to 60% of elderly patients are malnourished and an estimated 22% to 28% are at nutritional risk. In comparison with other health care settings, there is limited literature on the prevalence of malnutrition in community-dwelling older adults, especially in the prefrail/frail older population. However, the reported prevalence indicates a range of 5% to 30%.[10] Data from the Geriatric Frailty Clinic for Assessment of Frailty and Prevention of Disability showed that 8% of prefrail/frail older people experienced malnutrition; a risk of malnutrition concerned 39.5%.[11] In the residential aged care setting, the reported PEM prevalence ranges from 16% to 70% depending on the assessment tool used and the level of care required.[10]

In summary, the prevalence of PEM increases with age. It is 5% to 30% in elderly persons living at home, 16% to 70% in those in institutional care, and 20% to 60% in hospitalized elderly patients.

RISK FACTORS OF MALNUTRITION IN ELDERLY

The cause of malnutrition in elderly is multifactorial. Aging is accompanied by physiologic changes that can negatively impact nutritional status: sensory impairment (decreased sense of taste and smell) may result in reduced appetite; poor oral health and dental problems can lead to difficulty chewing, inflammation, and a monotonous diet that is poor in quality; progressive loss of vision and hearing may also limit mobility and affect the elderly's ability to shop for food and prepare meals. Along with physiologic changes, the elderly may also experience profound psychosocial and environmental changes, such as isolation, loneliness, depression, and inadequate finances. These changes affect dietary intake ultimately impacting nutritional status. Finally, dementia is also associated with an increased risk of unintentional weight loss and malnutrition.

In conclusion, each of these factors must alert the health professional and close relatives. This is especially the case if several factors are combined. Moreover, many diseases may be accompanied by malnutrition because of anorexia. Anorexia is a frequent symptom in the elderly, and it is essential to systematically seek a cause.

CONSEQUENCES OF MALNUTRITION IN ELDERLY

It is well documented that older patients are known to be especially vulnerable to PEM-related consequences,[10] such as prolonged length of stay in hospital, increased risk of falls, admission to higher level care, decreased physical function, poorer quality of life, increased risk of life-threatening complications, and increased mortality. Pressure ulcers are twice as likely to develop in malnourished hospital patients compared with well-nourished patients, and the risk of surgical site infections is 3 times higher.[12]

Use of an inappropriate screening tool (one that has not been validated or has been validated in a different population) negatively influences patient care and risks misdiagnosis (or missed diagnosis) of nutrition-related problems.

In summary, in the elderly, malnutrition causes or worsens a state of frailty and/or dependency and contributes to the development of morbidities. It is also associated with a worsening of the prognosis of underlying diseases and increases the risk of death.

NUTRITION SCREENING

Nutrition screening is the recommended first step in the nutrition care process as it allows the early identification of nutritional concerns.[12,13] Given the multifactorial nature of malnutrition in the elderly, and in the absence of a single objective measure or gold standard, several nutrition screening tools specific to the older adult population have been developed. Well-known examples include MNA,[1–3] MST,[4] MUST,[5] NRS 2002,[6] SGA[7] and SNAQ.[8]

Nutrition screening and nutrition assessment are terms often used interchangeably in the literature and in practice despite their differences. The Academy of Nutrition and Dietetics defines *nutrition screening* as "the process of identifying patients, clients, or groups who may have a nutrition diagnosis and benefit from nutrition assessment and intervention by a registered dietitian."[14] Similarly, the American Society for Parenteral and Enteral Nutrition, an interdisciplinary organization whose members span the health care continuum (registered nurses, pharmacists, physicians, scientists, and other nutrition support health professionals) define *nutrition screening* as "a process to identify an individual who is malnourished or who is at risk for malnutrition to determine if a detailed nutrition assessment is indicated."[15] In contrast, the longer, more detailed nutrition assessment process identifies (diagnoses) a nutrition problem and its cause and recommends an intervention. An understanding of the cause helps to determine the most feasible and effective intervention to implement for resolution of the diagnosis. Simply, screening determines the risk of a problem (eg, MNA-Short Form [MNA-SF], MST, MUST, NRS 2002, SNAQ), and assessment determines the presence of a problem (eg, full MNA, SGA).[12]

Nutrition Screening Tools

Malnutrition screening tool

The MST instrument consists of 2 questions related to recent unintentional weight loss and eating poorly because of a decreased appetite.[2] The MST results in a score between 0 and 5, with patients considered to be at risk of malnutrition if they score 2 or greater. The MST has been validated in acute hospital and ambulatory care but not specifically in long-term-care settings.

Malnutrition university screening tool

The MUST is a universal tool designed for use across settings and consists of a body mass index (BMI) category (BMI <20 is indicated as at risk), a weight loss category (unintentional weight loss during the past 3 to 6 months), and an acute disease score.[5] A score of 1 indicates medium risk, and a score of 2 or more indicates a high malnutrition risk. MUST is recommended by the European Society for Parenteral and Enteral Nutrition (ESPEN) for screening adults in the community.

Nutritional risk screening 2002

The NRS 2002 has 3 components: (1) nutritional status, which incorporates 3 separate items: categories of BMI (<18.5, 18.5–20.5 [plus an additional item of impaired general condition for these two categories], and >20.5 kg/m^2), categories about weight loss (>5% in 3 months, >5% in 2 months, and >5% in 1 month [>15% in 3 months]), and the assessment of food intake as a proportion of the normal requirement in the preceding week (0%–25%, 25%–50%, 50%–75%, and >75%); (2) disease severity; and (3) age, with all patients aged 70 years and older being given an additional score. The total score can range from 0 to 7, with values of 3 or greater indicating a likelihood of benefit from nutritional intervention.[6] Unlike the MNA, which was developed for use in elderly people in and outside hospitals, and unlike the MUST, which was developed specifically for all care settings, including hospitals, the NRS 2002 was primarily developed and promoted for use in adults in the hospital setting. It aimed to establish a screening procedure that would relate to clinically relevant outcomes resulting from nutritional interventions.

Simplified nutritional assessment questionnaire

The SNAQ instrument consists of 4 items that have been found to be predictive of weight loss at 6 months in community-dwelling and long-term-care residents.[8] The SNAQ instrument asks questions regarding appetite, early satiety, food taste, and number of meals consumed daily, with a score of 14 or less indicating a significant risk of at least 5% weight loss within 6 months (Appendix 1).

Nutrition Assessment Tools

Subjective global assessment

The SGA is a valid and reliable tool for assessing nutritional status in older adults. The ESPEN recommends SGA as the optimal tool for further nutrition assessment.[7] The SGA instrument takes into consideration a resident's medical history (eg, weight loss, dietary intake, gastrointestinal symptoms, and functional capacity) and a physical examination (eg, subcutaneous fat, muscle wasting, and edema). Residents are assessed as well nourished (category A), moderately malnourished (category B), or severely malnourished (category C).

Mini nutritional assessment: a 2-step screening process

The MNA was originally developed to provide a simple, reliable way to screen the nutritional status of persons older than 65 years and to add a nutrition component to the Comprehensive Geriatric Assessment.[1–3] The full MNA consists of 18 questions (scoring 0–30) covering anthropometric assessment (eg, BMI, midarm circumference, and calf circumference), general assessment (eg, lives in nursing home, medications, dementia, and depression), dietary assessment (eg, eating a full meal, protein, and fruit and vegetable intake), and self-assessment (eg, how they rate their health status compared with people of similar age). It classifies one as normally nourished (24–30 points), at risk for malnutrition (17.0–23.5 points), or malnourished (<17 points). It was well validated in the hospital, community, and long-term-care settings.[1] To save time in screening, Rubenstein and colleagues[2] developed a shortened version, the MNA-SF, and created a 2-step screening process. Six questions with the strongest correlation on the original MNA comprised the MNA-SF. The short form (as well as the revised short form using the measure of the calf circumference instead of the BMI[3]) was validated in the ambulatory care setting as a quicker way to screen large groups of people and eliminated the need to complete the full MNA when a person was normally nourished. When the MNA-SF classified a person at risk (8–11 points), the full 18-question MNA had to be completed to determine if the person was truly malnourished. MNA is recommended by the ESPEN for screening elderly people.

Some tools incorporate BMI for detecting the risk of PEM. BMI is a simple index of weight for height (defined as weight in kilograms divide by the square of height in meters [kg/m^2]). Individuals are classified as underweight (BMI <18.5 kg/m^2), normal weight (18.5–24.9 kg/m^2), overweight (25.0–29.9 kg/m^2), or obese ($\geq$30.0 kg/m^2). The choice of BMI cutoff points to identify underweight can have a major influence on the prevalence of these conditions. The rationale for higher BMI cutoff points is that older adults are likely to (1) have a smaller proportion of lean body mass than younger adults (as a result of aging, PEM, or inactivity) and (2) shorten with age because of the compression associated with an osteoporotic spine (kyphosis).[16] A BMI lower than 21 kg/m^2 is a relevant cutoff to identify malnutrition among the older population.[17] This cutoff was included in screening tools, such as the MUST or MNA. In the United States, a BMI less than 18.5 kg/m^2 is generally used to screen undernourished older people.[18] If patients cannot stand upright or have a spine curvature problem (dorsal kyphosis), it is possible to use Chumlea's formulae to estimate height from the heel-knee height or use the self-reported height (**Box 1**). A BMI of 21 kg/m^2 or greater does not exclude a risk of malnutrition or PEM in normal weight, overweight (IMC $\geq$25 kg/m^2), or obese (IMC $\geq$30 kg/m^2) elderly patients. Many studies have

Box 1
Chumlea's formulae

- For women: H (cm) = 84.88 – 0.24 × age (years) + 1.83 × knee height (cm), where *H* is height
- For men: H (cm) = 64.19 – 0.04 × age (years) + 2.03 × knee height (cm), where *H* is height

Knee height is measured with patients lying on their back, knees bent at 90°, using a height caliper placed under the foot with the mobile blade placed above the knee, at the condyles.

reported an increased prevalence of obese people living in nursing homes. In France, 18% of residents are obese within 12% experienced a weight loss at the time of initial assessment.[19]

According to the guidelines produced by the French General Directorate of Health,[13] "screening for malnutrition is recommended in all elderly subjects and must be carried out at least once a year in general practice, on admission and then once monthly in institutions, and during each hospital stay. Elderly persons at risk of malnutrition should be screened more frequently, according to the subject's clinical status and the degree of risk."[13] Screening for malnutrition is based on a search for risk factors of malnutrition, estimation of appetite and/or food intake, measurement of body weight, evaluation of weight loss compared with a previous record, and calculation of BMI. Screening may use a questionnaire including at least a search for risk factors and body weight changes, such as the MNA.[1–3] Any weight loss is a warning sign of malnutrition. Elderly persons should be weighed in general practice, at each visit; in an institution, on admission, then at least once monthly; in the hospital on admission, then at least once weekly during a short stay, every 15 days for rehabilitation care, and once monthly during long-term care. The diagnosis of malnutrition is based on the presence of one or more of the following criteria[13]:

- *Weight loss of 5% or greater in 1 month or 10% or greater in 6 months*: Ideally the reference weight is obtained from an earlier medical record. If it is not available, the usual self-reported body weight may be used. In the case of acute illness, the body weight must be that measured before the onset of the disorder. Factors that may influence the interpretation of the result, such as dehydration, edema, or fluid effusions, should be taken into account.
- *BMI* less than *21 kg/m*^{2}
- *Serum albumin concentrations* less than *35 g/L*: Hypoalbuminemia is not specific to malnutrition and may be observed in many disorders independent of nutritional status, in particular during inflammatory processes. The serum albumin assay result should, therefore, be interpreted after taking into account the inflammatory status evaluated by assay of C-reactive protein. Serum albumin concentration is a major prognostic factor of morbidity and mortality. Moreover, it may be used to distinguish 2 forms of malnutrition: (1) malnutrition caused by an isolated deficiency in food intake in which serum albumin may be normal and (2) malnutrition associated with inflammation and hypercatabolism during which there is a rapid fall in serum albumin levels.
- *Full MNA score* less than *17*

It is important to distinguish severe forms of malnutrition (weight loss $\geq$10% in 1 month or $\geq$15% in 6 months, BMI <18 kg/m^2, serum albumin <30 g/L). These forms are associated with a considerable increase in morbidity and mortality and, therefore, require rapid nutritional management.

In conclusion, given the high prevalence of malnutrition and lack of proper management of patients in various settings, performing a routine nutritional screening should result in early identification of patients who might have otherwise been missed. The nutritional support strategy is based on the patients' nutritional status and on the spontaneous food energy and protein intake. It must also take into account the nature and severity of any underlying diseases and associated disabilities as well as their foreseeable outcome (swallowing disorders for example). In French guidelines,[13] the objective of nutritional support in malnourished elderly patients is to achieve an energy intake of from 30 to 40 kcal/kg/d and a protein intake of from 1.2 to 1.5 g of protein per kilogram per day. The nutritional requirements will vary among patients and according to the disease background. Support must also integrate the opinion of patients and their close relatives as well as ethical considerations. Apart from situations contraindicating oral feeding, nutritional support should, as a priority, be initiated by providing dietary advice and/or fortified foods, if possible in collaboration with a dietician. Oral nutritional supplementation may be given if these supportive measures are ineffective or from the outset in patients with severe malnutrition. Enteral nutrition may be attempted if it impossible to achieve adequate oral nutritional support.

The various treatable causes of weight loss are easily remembered by the mnemonic MEALS-ON-WHEELS proposed by J. Morley (Appendix 2).[20]

Parenteral nutrition is restricted to the 3 following situations: (1) severe anatomic or functional malabsorption syndromes, (2) acute or chronic bowel obstruction, and (3) failure of well-conducted enteral nutrition (poor tolerability). It should be implemented in specialized departments within the scope of a coherent treatment plan.

REFERENCES

1. Vellas B, Villars H, Abellan G, et al. Overview of the MNA-Its history and challenges. J Nutr Health Aging 2006;10(6):456–63.
2. Rubenstein LZ, Harker JO, Salvà A, et al. Screening for undernutrition in geriatric practice: developing the short-form mini-nutritional assessment (MNA-SF). J Gerontol A Biol Sci Med Sci 2001,56(6).M366–72.
3. Kaiser MJ, Bauer JM, Ramsch C, et al, MNA-International Group. Validation of the Mini Nutritional Assessment short-form (MNA-SF): a practical tool for identification of nutritional status. J Nutr Health Aging 2009;13(9):782–8.
4. Ferguson M, Capra S, Bauer J, et al. Development of a valid and reliable malnutrition screening tool for adult acute hospital patients. Nutrition 1999;15(6): 458–64.
5. Stratton RJ, Hackston A, Longmore D, et al. Malnutrition in hospital outpatients and inpatients: prevalence, concurrent validity and ease of use of the 'malnutrition universal screening tool' ('MUST') for adults. Br J Nutr 2004;92: 799–808.
6. Kondrup J, Rasmussen HH, Hamberg O, et al, Ad hoc EsPEN working group. Nutritional risk screening (NRs 2002): a new method based on an analysis of controlled clinical trials. Clin Nutr 2003;22:321–36.
7. Detsky AS, McLaughlin JR, Baker JP, et al. What is subjective global assessment of nutritional status? JPEN J Parenter Enteral Nutr 1987;11(1):8–13.
8. Wilson MM, Thomas DR, Rubenstein LZ, et al. Appetite assessment: simple appetite questionnaire predicts weight loss in community-dwelling adults and nursing home residents. Am J Clin Nutr 2005;82(5):1074–81.
9. Fried LP, Tangen CM, Walston J, et al. Frailty in older adults: evidence for a phenotype. J Gerontol A Biol Sci Med Sci 2001;56:M146–56.
10. Agarwal E, Miller M, Yaxley A, et al. Malnutrition in the elderly: a narrative review. Maturitas 2013;76:296–302.
11. Tavassoli N, Guyonnet S, Abellan Van Kan G. Descritpion of 1108 older patients referred by their physician to the "Geriatric Frailty Clinic (GFC) for assessment of frailty and prevention of disability" at the Gerontopole. J Nutr Health Aging 2014; 18(5):457–64.

12. Field L, Hand R. Differentiating malnutrition screening and assessment: a nutrition care process perspective. J Acad Nutr Diet 2015;115(5):824–8.
13. Available at: http://www.has-sante.fr/portail/upload/docs/application/pdf/denutrition_personne_agee_2007_-_recommandations.pdf Janvier 2015.
14. Academy of Nutrition and Dietetics. Definitions and criteria. Nutrition Screening Evidence Analysis Project. 2014. Available at: http://and evidencelibrary.com/topic.cfm?cat=3958.
15. American Society for Parenteral and Enteral Nutrition (APSEN). Board of Directors and Clinical Practice Committee. Definitions of terms, styles, and conventions used in APSEN. Board of Directors approved documents. 2010. Available at: http://www.nutritioncare.org/Clinical_Practice_Library/.
16. Elia M, Stratton RJ. An analytic appraisal of nutrition screening tools supported by original data with particular reference to age. Nutrition 2012;28:477–94.
17. Sergi G, Perissinotto E, Pisent C, et al. An adequate threshold for body mass index to detect underweight condition in elderly persons: the Italian Longitudinal Study on Aging (ILSA). J Gerontol A Biol Sci Med Sci 2005;60(7):866–71.
18. Challa S, Sharkey JR, Chen M, et al. Association of resident, facility, and geographic characteristics with chronic undernutrition in a nationally represented sample of older residents in U.S. nursing homes. J Nutr Health Aging 2007;11:179–84.
19. Zanandrea V, Barreto de Souto P, Cesari M, et al. Obesity and nursing home: a review and an update. Clin Nutr 2013;32(5):679–85.
20. Morley JE. Undernutrition in older adults. Fam Pract 2012;29:89–93.

APPENDIX 1: THE SNAQ: A SCREENING TEST FOR ANOREXIA

1. My appetite is
   - A. Very poor
   - B. Poor
   - C. Average
   - D. Good
   - E. Very good
2. When I eat
   - A. I feel full after eating only a few mouthfuls
   - B. I feel full after eating about a third of a meal
   - C. I feel full after eating more than half a meal
   - D. I feel full after eating most of the meal
   - E. I hardly ever feel full
3. Food tastes
   - A. Very bad
   - B. Bad
   - C. Average
   - D. Good
   - E. Very good

4. Normally I eat
   A. Less than one meal a day
   B. One meal a day
   C. Two meals a day
   D. Three meals a day
   E. More than 3 meals a day

Instructions: Complete the questionnaire by circling the correct answers and then tally the results based on the following numerical scale: A = 1, B = 2, C = 3, D = 4, E = 5.

Scoring: If the score is less than 14, there is a significant risk of weight loss.

From Wilson MM, Thomas DR, Rubenstein LZ, et al. Appetite assessment: simple appetite questionnaire predicts weight loss in community-dwelling adults and nursing home residents. Am J Clin Nutr 2005;82(5):1074–81; with permission.

APPENDIX 2: MEALS-ON-WHEELS: MNEMONIC AS AN EASY METHOD TO SCREEN FOR CAUSES OF WEIGHT LOSS IN OLDER PERSONS

*M*edications (eg, digoxin, theophylline, cimetidine)

*E*motional (eg, depression)

*A*lcoholism, elder abuse, anorexia tardive

*L*ate-life paranoia

*S*wallowing problems

*O*ral factors

*N*osocomial infections (eg, tuberculosis)

*W*andering and other dementia-related factors

*H*yperthyroidism, hypercalcemia, hypoadrenalism

*E*nteral problems (eg, gluten enteropathy)

*E*ating problems

*L*ow-salt, low-cholesterol, and other therapeutic diets

*S*tones (cholecystitis)

From Morley JE. Undernutrition in older adults. Fam Pract 2012;29:89–93; with permission.

Diabetes, Nutrition, and Exercise

Ahmed H. Abdelhafiz, MSc, MD, FRCP[a], Alan J. Sinclair, MSc, MD, FRCP[b,*]

KEYWORDS

• Aging • Diabetes • Sarcopenia • Nutrition • Exercise

KEY POINTS

- The prevalence of diabetes is increasing, especially in older people because of increased life expectancy.
- Aging is associated with body composition changes, with increased visceral fat and reduced muscle mass or sarcopenia increasing insulin resistance.
- The increased prevalence of sarcopenia and undernutrition in old age are associated with the characteristic diabetes phenotype in old age of frailty and disability.
- Because of the age-related body composition changes, the potential benefits of nutrition and exercise intervention in older people with diabetes are enormous.

INTRODUCTION

With increasing aging of the population and urbanization of lifestyle, the prevalence of diabetes is likely to reach epidemic levels in most countries, especially in older people more than 75 years of age.[1] Aging is associated with body composition changes that lead to insulin resistance, glucose intolerance, and increased risk of diabetes.[2] As a result, diabetes is increasingly becoming a disease of old age.

Diabetes in old age is a disabling disease because of the traditionally associated vascular complications, coexisting morbidities, and the increased prevalence of geriatric syndromes and frailty. Because obesity and physical inactivity are associated with type 2 diabetes,[3] weight loss to achieve optimal body weight and exercise training are the cornerstones of prevention and treatment. Although diabetes may be associated with obesity in some older people, underweight is also common, especially among those living in care homes. Both conditions may signify inadequate nutritional status or malnutrition. Therefore, achieving optimal body weight is less straightforward and needs to be individualized because of the heterogeneity in this

[a] Department of Elderly Medicine, Rotherham General Hospital, Moorgate Road, Rotherham S60 2UD, UK; [b] Foundation for Diabetes Research in Older People, Diabetes Frail Ltd, Droitwich Spa WR9 0QH, UK
* Corresponding author.
E-mail address: sinclair.5@btinternet.com

Clin Geriatr Med 31 (2015) 439–451
http://dx.doi.org/10.1016/j.cger.2015.04.011 geriatric.theclinics.com
0749-0690/15/$ – see front matter

age group. Exercise training also increases insulin sensitivity and muscle mass, and improves glycemic control; however, the benefits of exercise and the potential of exercise prescription are still underused.[4] The aim of diabetes management in older people is to slow progression of the disease, prevent the development of complications, maintain independency, and improve quality of life through a combination of adequate nutrition, exercise, and medications. Good nutritional status and good functional capacity have been shown to be associated with good quality of life in older people with type 2 diabetes.[5] This article reviews the diabetogenic effects of aging, diabetes phenotype in old age, and lifestyle modifications through nutrition and exercise in older people with diabetes.

EPIDEMIOLOGY

The worldwide prevalence of diabetes is increasing and will double from the year 2000 to 2030, with the greatest increase in people more than 65 years of age.[6] In France, the prevalence increased with age to 14.2% in those aged 65 to 74 years, peaking at 19.7% in men and 14.2% in women aged 75 to 79 years.[7] In the United States, total diabetes prevalence is estimated to be 14% of the population and is highest in those aged 65 years or older and by the year 2050 diabetes prevalence could be as high as 33%.[8] The burden of diabetes is likely to grow faster in the low and middle income countries, probably because of aging of the population and urbanization associated with lifestyle change. The prevalence of diabetes among older Chinese in rural Taiwan was 16.9% in 2000, mean (standard deviation [SD]) age 72.6 (6) years at baseline, and increased to 23.7% in 2005.[9] In minority ethnic groups living in the developed world, the prevalence of diabetes is higher than in white populations. For example, the prevalence of diabetes in older (≥75 years) Mexican American adults almost doubled between 1993 to 1994 and 2004 to 2005, from 20.3% to 37.2%, respectively, compared with the increase in the general population of the same age group from 10.4% to 16.4%.[10] The prevalence of diabetes among African Americans and Hispanic people has consistently been higher than among white people and is projected to triple by the year 2050 and only to double in white people. The prevalence of diabetes in care homes is higher than in the community. In the United States, around 24.6% of nursing home residents had diabetes in 2004. Among residents aged 65 to 74, 75 to 84, and greater than or equal to 85 years, diabetes prevalence was 36.1%, 29.5%, and 18.3%, respectively.[11] There was a steady increase in the prevalence of diabetes between 1995 and 2004, from 16.3% to 23.4%, with an average change of 0.8% per year. A more recent survey showed a further increase in the prevalence of diabetes affecting 32.8% of residents of nursing homes.[12] Ethnic disparities in diabetes prevalence are also well documented in care home settings. The odds of diabetes are about 2 times higher in black and Hispanic residents relative to white residents, and diabetes was present in 22.5% and 35.6% of white people and nonwhite people respectively.[11]

DIABETOGENIC EFFECTS OF AGING

Normal glucose homeostasis requires both normal insulin secretion by the beta cells of the pancreas and normal peripheral glucose use by peripheral tissues that are sensitive to insulin. Aging is associated with changes in body fat distribution with a reduction in subcutaneous fat and increase in visceral fat, which is linked to increased insulin resistance.[13] Visceral fat accumulation with aging leads to altered lipid metabolism with increased rate of lipolysis producing high levels of free fatty acids, which may have a role in reducing peripheral insulin sensitivity.[14] Muscle mass declines with aging because of physical inactivity and, because the muscle tissue is the main site of glucose consumption, the loss of muscle mass also increases insulin resistance.[15] Accumulation of lipids within the muscles and reduced mitochondrial function are other factors leading to insulin resistance.[16] Aging is associated with a reduction in insulin secretion by 0.7% per year caused by a combination of beta-cell dysfunction and increased beta-cell apoptosis, and individuals with glucose intolerance show a 50% reduction in beta-cell mass.[17] Beta-cell autoimmunity may lead to activation of acute phase response in older people with diabetes.[18] In genetically predisposed individuals, long-term hypersecretion of interleukins, C-reactive protein, and tumor necrosis factor alpha may contribute to impaired beta-cell insulin secretion and insulin resistance.[18] Therefore, the diabetogenic effects of aging are related to increased insulin resistance and reduced insulin secretion. It is possible that insulin resistance develops in the prediabetes state and beta cells compensate by increasing insulin secretion, causing hyperinsulinemia and initially maintaining normal glucose tolerance. Eventually, because of a combination of reduced insulin secretory capacity of beta cells to compensate for insulin resistance and further diminution of peripheral tissue sensitivity to insulin, insulin secretion becomes inadequate, leading to the progression to persistent hyperglycemia, glucose intolerance, and then to diabetes (**Box 1**).

DIABETES PHENOTYPE IN OLD AGE

Older people with diabetes are exposed to the interplay between metabolic dysfunction, vascular disease, and the aging process in combination with other age-related disorders. Diabetes phenotype in old age is characterized by the associated comorbidity burden and geriatric syndromes such as cognitive dysfunction, depression, falls, and incontinence. This complex phenotype may lead to malnutrition and physical inactivity and eventually the development of frailty and disability, which have a direct

Box 1
Diabetogenic effects and diabetes phenotype of aging

Diabetogenic effects (increased insulin resistance and decreased insulin secretion)

- Increased visceral body fat
- Reduced skeletal muscle mass
- Decreased beta-cell function
- Reduced beta-cell mass
- Mitochondrial dysfunction
- Increased inflammatory markers
- Altered lipid metabolism

Diabetes phenotype (frailty and disability)

- Multiple comorbidities
- Geriatric syndromes
- Physical inactivity
- Malnutrition
- Sarcopenia
- Poor muscle quality
- Weight loss

impact on diabetes management by lifestyle modification through nutrition and exercise training interventions.

Frailty

Frailty is a condition characterized by a reduction in physiologic reserve and in the ability to resist physical or psychological stressors.[19] Its definition is largely based on the presence of 3 or more phenotypes (weight loss, weakness, decreased physical activity, exhaustion, and slow gait speed).[20] Frailty is considered to be a wasting disease with weight loss being one of its criteria. Undernutrition, which is very common in older people, seems to be a risk factor for frailty. In the United States, about 16% of elderly persons living in the community are undernourished. These figures increase to 59% in long-term care institutions and 65% in acute-care hospitals.[21] Sarcopenia or muscle mass loss is a component of frailty that seems to be accelerated when diabetes is present. In a community study of 3153 participants greater than or equal to 65 years of age, appendicular lean mass loss in men with diabetes was twice that of men without diabetes (3.0% vs 1.5%) and in women with diabetes was 1.8 times that of those without diabetes (3.4% vs 1.9%) over 4 years of follow up. The mechanisms explaining these results may be related to reduced muscle protein synthesis caused by lower testosterone and insulinlike growth factor 1 levels and increased muscle protein breakdown caused by a higher rate of inflammation.[22] Diabetes also causes sarcopenia because of the catabolic effect of insulin deficiency and by increasing intramyocellular lipid accumulation.[23] In another study, older persons with type 2 diabetes had accelerated decline in leg lean mass, muscle strength, and longer sit-to-stand time compared with normoglycemic control subjects.[24] Other factors of malnutrition and frailty may be related to the oral health of older people with diabetes. For example, optimal nutrition may not be maintained because of poor dentition, a dry mouth, reduced taste sensation and palatability, and appetite change with increasing age.[25]

Disability

Aging and diabetes are associated with mobility decline and physical inactivity.

Development of frailty leads to a decline in function and eventual disability. It has been shown that about 28% of older people with diabetes require some help with activities of daily living compared with only 16% of those without diabetes, and only half of the cases of functional decline were explained by the traditional complications of diabetes, such as coronary artery disease, stroke, and peripheral vascular disease. The unexplained worsening in function could be caused by muscle weakness and frailty.[26] Diabetes is associated with a 2-fold increased risk of being unable to perform daily physical tasks such as walking, doing house work, or climbing stairs, and 1.6-fold greater risk of difficulties performing basic personal care such as bathing, using the toilet, dressing, and eating.[27] Diabetes complications such as neuropathy, arthritis, and vascular disease are contributors to physical disability in older people with diabetes.[28] The Study of Osteoporotic Fractures has shown that diabetes also increases the risk of falls (odds ratio, 2.78; 95% confidence interval, 1.82–4.25). History of arthritis, musculoskeletal pain, depression, poor vision, and peripheral neuropathy are the main predictors of falling among older people with diabetes (see **Box 1**).[29]

LIFESTYLE MODIFICATIONS

Because age-related body composition changes lead to reduced muscle mass and insulin resistance and diabetes phenotype in old age is associated with both malnutrition leading to frailty and physical inactivity leading to disability, older people with diabetes potentially benefit most from lifestyle modifications through nutrition and exercise training interventions.

NUTRITION

The goal of nutritional therapy is to maintain a good metabolic profile and achieve optimum body weight. A diet that is high in fiber and potassium and low in saturated fats and refined carbohydrates and salt, in addition to achievement of ideal body weight, improves the lipid profile, significantly decreases blood pressure, and reduces the overall cardiovascular risk.[30] Diet should be sufficient in micronutrients such as phosphate, chromium, and zinc for adequate metabolism and insulin action. It would ideally be consistent in volumes of carbohydrate at each mealtime with a preference for low glycemic index choices and no concentrated sweets to help avoid food-related postprandial hyperglycemia. To minimize the risk of hypoglycemia, additional carbohydrates should be taken before or during exercise, with immediate access to a source of rapidly absorbed carbohydrate in case hypoglycemia occurs. A healthy diet has a role in reducing the incidence of diabetes and improving glycemic control. In the Diabetes Prevention Program, lifestyle intervention, including modest weight reduction, a healthy low-fat diet, and regular exercise, reduced the development of diabetes in older people and this beneficial effect persisted for up to 10 years after the end of the study.[31] Muscle mass is important for blood glucose homeostasis because increased muscle volume can increase insulin sensitivity and blood glucose uptake. Muscle mass depends on a balance between muscle protein synthesis and breakdown. Sarcopenia or frailty in old age occurs as a result of a gradual net loss of skeletal muscle protein. In older people there is diminished muscle protein synthesis in response to anabolic stimuli such as protein ingestion compared with younger people.[32] Therefore, older people in general need more dietary proteins than do younger people to compensate for this age-related anabolic resistance. They may also need more protein to offset inflammatory and catabolic conditions associated with the chronic and acute diseases that occur commonly with aging. An average daily intake in the range of 1.0 to 1.2 g protein per kilogram of body weight is recommended to help maintain lean body mass and function. Higher protein intake (1.2–1.5 g/kg body weight daily) is advised for people who are exercising or who have acute illness, with the exception of those with severe kidney disease (glomerular filtration rate <30 mL/min/1.73 m^2), who may need to limit their intake (0.8 g/kg body weight daily), although the renal benefit of a low-protein diet may increase the risk of malnutrition.[33,34] People with severe illness or marked malnutrition may need as much as 2.0 g/kg body weight per day.[33] Diabetes is associated with a faster loss of muscle strength and sarcopenic obesity. Therefore increased dietary protein intake may be of benefit. Older people with diabetes and no kidney disease can safely have up to 20% of their total energy as protein. Little research is available about the safety of higher protein (>20% of daily energy) diet. However, a recent study of older people, up to the age of 75 years, with diabetes but no kidney disease showed that those who had a high-protein diet (30% of daily energy) required 8% fewer hypoglycemic medications after 1 year compared with their baseline medications.[35] Anabolic resistance to protein feeding in older people could also be overcome by providing sufficient amounts of rapidly digested proteins rich in the essential amino acid leucine, such as whey protein, which may offset muscle loss and reduce sarcopenia.[36] Essential amino acids, in particular leucine, are primarily responsible for the amino acid stimulation of muscle protein anabolism in healthy older people and in initiating molecular events associated with muscle hypertrophy promoting positive muscle protein balance.[37] The increased intake of omega-3 fatty acids may help preserve muscle mass by relieving the anabolic resistance.[38] Older people with diabetes benefit from nutrition education designed to improve knowledge and skills to make healthy choices about their diet.[39] Decisions around nutrition should involve patients and their carers, taking into account individual circumstances and cultural and ethnic preferences (**Box 2**).

EXERCISE

Aging is associated with increased insulin resistance leading to the loss of skeletal muscle mass by reducing the normal anabolic effects of insulin on skeletal muscle protein synthesis stimulation and breakdown inhibition.[40] In addition to the aging effect, diabetes induces a greater muscle mass loss, worse muscle quality (defined as muscle strength per unit of muscle mass), reduced upper and lower body strength, and greater visceral fat content.[41] It has been shown that older people with diabetes, mean (SD) age 71 (1) years, have accelerated decline in leg lean mass, muscle strength, and functional capacity compared with individuals without diabetes.[24] Therefore, exercise training is an important part of diabetes prevention and management to improve body composition, insulin resistance, glucose control, and overall function. The 2 common types of exercise are aerobic exercise, which recruits large groups of muscles and includes activities such as walking, cycling, swimming, or jogging, and, resistance exercise, which uses muscular strength to lift a weight or to move a load, causing isolated and brief activity of a single muscle group (**Table 1**). Aerobic exercise may not be suitable for all older people because of the high prevalence of comorbidities such as arthritis, cardiovascular disease, peripheral vascular disease, neuropathy, and poor mobility. Resistance exercise may be a safer alternative for these patients. It has been suggested that there is no evidence that differences between aerobic and resistance exercises are of clinical importance. There is also no evidence that resistance exercise differs from aerobic exercise in its impact on cardiovascular risk markers or safety.[42] Resistance training has been shown to improve muscle quality, resulting in skeletal muscle fiber hypertrophy in addition to

Box 2
Goals of nutrition and exercise in older people with diabetes

- To maintain good metabolic profile
- Maintenance of healthy body weight
- Avoidance of malnutrition
- Maintenance of skeletal muscle mass
- Maintenance of hydration
- To address individual needs based on personal and cultural preferences
- Improve body composition with reduced visceral fat
- Reduce insulin resistance
- Improve muscle quality
- Improve overall physical function
- Maintain good quality of life

Table 1
Comparison of aerobic and resistance exercise

	Aerobic	Resistance
Muscles involved	Large groups of muscle contracting continuously	One group of muscle contracting intermittently
Examples	Walking and jogging	Lifting or moving load
Metabolic effects		
Improved insulin sensitivity	++	++
Increase glucose uptake	++	++
Improves lipid profile	++	++
Blood pressure control	++	++
Improves aerobic capacity	+++	+
Body composition effects		
Reduction of body fats	++	+
Increase muscle mass	+	+++
Increase muscle strength	+	+++
Duration	Long	Short
Suitability	Reasonably fit persons	Persons with comorbidities or poor mobility
Overall improvement	Improves stamina	Improves force

improvement in biochemical markers that increase insulin sensitivity in older Hispanic people (mean [SD] age 66.0 [2] years) with diabetes.[43] In a systematic review of 372 participants with type 2 diabetes, average age 58.4 years (range, 46.5–67.6 years), progressive resistance training (PRT) exercise, defined as exercise in which the resistance against which a muscle generates force is progressively increased over time, led to a significant reduction of hemoglobin A1c (HbA1c) (0.3%) compared with no exercise but was similar to aerobic exercise. PRT resulted in improvements in strength compared with aerobic or no exercise. Eight weeks with 2 to 3 sessions of 45 minutes' duration of PRT exercise was sufficient to produce improvements in glycemic control.[44] In a systematic review of PRT in older people with diabetes, PRT generally had an effect on the musculoskeletal system, disease process, and body composition to varying degrees. Overall, PRT had the largest effect on the musculoskeletal measures (muscle size, strength, and quality defined as strength per unit of muscle mass), especially lower body muscles, followed by disease process measures (glycemic control and metabolic profile), whereas the smallest effect was seen on the body composition measures (body fat).[45] A combination of both exercise modalities may be optimal. In a study of 136 sedentary and abdominally obese older people with diabetes, mean (SD) age 67.7 (5.1) years, the combination of resistance (60 minutes) and aerobic (90 minutes) exercise, performed across 3 days per week was the optimal exercise strategy for simultaneous reduction in insulin resistance and improvement in function. Improvement in insulin resistance was mainly driven by the aerobic exercise, whereas improvement in function was driven by resistance exercise. Reduction of visceral fat and increase in muscle mass may respectively explain the improvement in insulin resistance and function.[46] The choice of exercise type for older people with diabetes may be decided according to comorbidities, personal preference, or available resources. Using one or the other type of exercise may be less important than doing some form of physical activity (see **Box 2**).

NUTRITION-EXERCISE INTERACTION

Protein intake along with exercise training synergistically increases skeletal muscle mass. Exercise helps to reduce muscle protein breakdown and increases muscle protein synthesis. Protein intake results in an increased availability of amino acids, especially the essential amino acid leucine, which promotes a net inward gradient for amino acid transport to the intracellular free amino acid pool, providing the signal and building blocks for the stimulation of muscle protein synthesis. Therefore, periodic feeding induces shifts in the net protein balance from negative during fasting to positive after feeding. Combining the exercise-induced and feeding-induced increase in muscle protein synthesis results in periodic increases in accretion of proteins and eventually muscle hypertrophy. Protein ingestion at intervals over 24 hours after exercise, as opposed to 1 large protein meal, may be able to elicit a potent anabolic response in older people and promote muscle protein accretion for hypertrophy.[47] It has been shown that protein supplementation for frail older people who were engaged in resistance training resulted in muscle hypertrophy, and increase in muscle strength, muscle mass, and performance.[48] Also the combination of diet quality and physical activity was associated with maintenance of muscle strength in older Australian men (aged 67–84 years) with diabetes but diet quality alone was not enough to preserve muscle strength in a secondary analysis of the longitudinal observational NuAge study.[49] The nutrition-exercise interaction is equally useful in overweight or obese individuals (predominantly through weight loss) as well as frail individuals (predominantly through increasing muscle mass) (**Fig. 1**).

Overweight

The synergistic effects of nutrition and exercise can play an important role in diabetes prevention and glucose control. The incidence of diabetes was 58% and 39% lower in

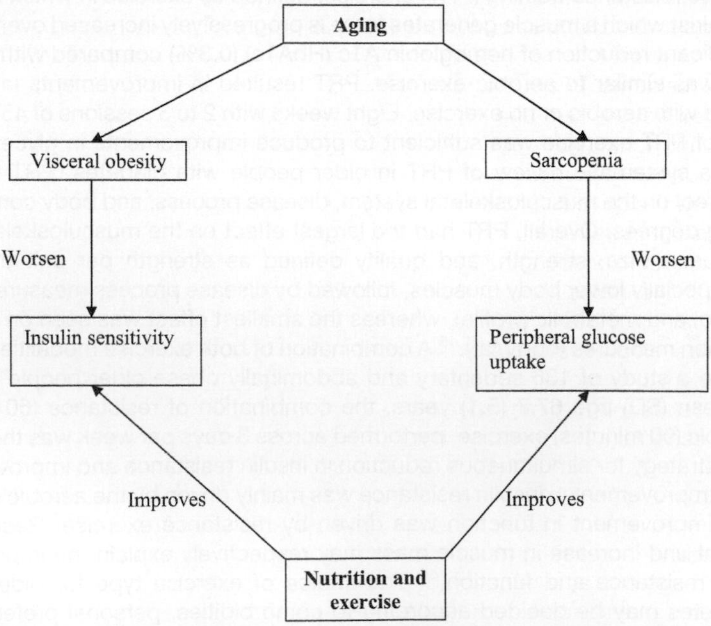

Fig. 1. Diabetogenic effects of aging and the beneficial effects of nutrition-exercise intervention.

individuals treated with intensive diet and exercise intervention compared with placebo or metformin respectively in the Diabetes Prevention Program.[50] Continued behavioral changes designed to promote and maintain weight loss through caloric restriction and increased physical activity compared with usual care in 1053 older (65–76 years) and 4092 younger (45–64 years) people with diabetes showed that older individuals had greater weight loss (6.2%) than younger participants (5.1%). There was a comparable increase in fitness and high-density lipoprotein cholesterol level and a decrease in HbA1c level and waist circumference over 4 years in both old and young intervention individuals compared with the usual care group. This finding suggests that intensive lifestyle intervention targeting weight loss and increased physical activity is effective in overweight and obese older individuals to produce sustained weight loss and improvements in fitness and cardiovascular risk factors.[51] Additional benefits of nutrition and exercise intervention for older people include improved walking balance. The Look AHEAD (Action for Health in Diabetes) study in middle-aged and older people with type 2 diabetes showed that weight loss and improved fitness decreased the risk for loss of mobility.[52] Reducing fats and simple carbohydrates content from the diet of obese individuals, rather than reducing the protein or the complex carbohydrates, combined with increasing physical activity are the goals for weight reduction without losing lean muscle mass.

Frail

In a study of the very elderly (mean [SD] age 87.1 [0.6] years), nursing home residents randomized to PRT, nutritional supplementation, both interventions, and neither, PRT was effective in reducing muscle loss but nutritional supplementation without concomitant exercise did not reduce muscle weakness. The positive effects of PRT were accompanied by better mobility. Improvements in muscle strength, gait velocity, stair climbing power, and spontaneous physical activity occurred in the exercise group but not in the nutritional supplementation alone group. This finding suggests that nutritional supplementation alone, without exercise, is not enough to keep muscle mass and preserve physical function.[53] Exercise in care homes seems feasible despite the frail nature of residents. In a systematic review of 13 studies of PRT in nursing home residents aged between 80 and 89 years, significant improvements occurred in muscle strength and functional performance outcomes, including chair-to-stand time, stair climbing, gait speed, balance, and functional capacity.[54] The proposed MID-Frail study will evaluate the clinical, functional, social, and economic impacts of a multimodal intervention (resistance training exercise, diet, and education) in frail and prefrail subjects aged greater than or equal to 70 years with type 2 diabetes compared with usual clinical practice.[55] The imposition of carbohydrate restrictions on frail older people with diabetes, especially those living in care homes, is not warranted. Malnutrition and dehydration may develop because of unnecessary restrictions. A liberalized diet for diabetes management to improve nutritional status without affecting glycemic control is suitable for frail older people. Maintenance of adequate hydration is another important aspect to monitor, especially in patients with cognitive impairment.

SUMMARY

The worldwide prevalence of diabetes is increasing with increasing age. With increasing age and accumulation of comorbidities and geriatric syndromes, diabetes phenotype in older people is characterized by sarcopenic obesity leading to frailty and disability. Sarcopenia or reduced muscle mass and obesity, mainly visceral, play a role in increasing insulin resistance and reducing peripheral blood glucose uptake, increasing the risk of developing diabetes or worsening glycemic control in older people with diabetes. Therefore, the potential benefits of nutrition and exercise training for older people with diabetes are enormous. Muscle mass loss is the result of a net negative muscle protein balance caused by imbalance between muscle protein synthesis and muscle protein breakdown. A good supplement of protein (especially the essential amino acid leucine), complex carbohydrates, and low saturated fat intake combined with exercise training acts as a strong stimulus for protein synthesis, producing a net positive protein balance and muscle hypertrophy, improving insulin sensitivity and overall physical function. Exercise training is feasible in older people, even in those living in care homes. The choice of exercise or diet type may be decided according to the prevalent comorbidities or available resources, involving patients and their carers and taking into account individual circumstances, and cultural and ethnic preferences.

REFERENCES

1. Cowie C, Rust KF, Ford ES, et al. Full accounting of diabetes and pre-diabetes in the U.S. population in 1988–1994 and 2005–2006. Diabetes Care 2009;32:287–94.
2. Meneilly GS, Tessier D. Diabetes in elderly adults. J Gerontol A Biol Sci Med Sci 2001;56:M5–13.
3. Beaufrere B, Morio B. Fat and protein redistribution with aging: metabolic considerations. Eur J Clin Nutr 2000;54(Suppl 3):S48–53.
4. Hordern MD, Dunstan DW, Prins JB, et al. Exercise prescription for patients with type 2 diabetes and pre-diabetes: a position statement from exercise and sport science Australia. J Sci Med Sport 2011;15:25–31.
5. Alfonso-Rosa RM, Pozo-Cruz BD, Pozo-Cruz JD, et al. The relationship between nutritional status, functional capacity, and health-related quality of life in older adults with type 2 diabetes: a pilot explanatory study. J Nutr Health Aging 2013;17:315–21.
6. Wild S, Roglic G, Green A, et al. Global prevalence of diabetes: estimates for the year 2000 and projections for 2030. Diabetes Care 2004;27:1047–53.
7. Ricci P, Blotière PO, Weill A, et al. Diabète traité en France: quelles évolutions entre 2000 et 2009? Bull Epidemiol Hebd (Paris) 2010;43:425–31.
8. Boyle JP, Thompson TJ, Gregg EW, et al. Projection of the year 2050 burden of diabetes in the US adult population: dynamic modeling of incidence, mortality, and prediabetes prevalence. Popul Health Metr 2010;8(1):29.
9. Li-Ning P, Ming-Hsien L, Hsiu-Yun L, et al. Risk factors of new onset diabetes mellitus among elderly Chinese in rural Taiwan. Age Ageing 2010;39:125–8.
10. Beard HA, Al Ghatrif M, Samper-Terent R, et al. Trends in diabetes prevalence and diabetes-related complications in older Mexican Americans from 1993–1994 to 2004–2005. Diabetes Care 2009;32:2212–7.
11. Resnick HE, Heineman J, Stone R, et al. Diabetes in U.S. nursing homes. Diabetes Care 2004;2008(31):287–8.
12. Dybicz SB, Thompson S, Molotsky S, et al. Prevalence of diabetes and the burden of comorbid conditions among elderly nursing home residents. Am J Geriatr Pharmacother 2011;9:212–23.
13. Kuk JL, Saunders TJ, Davidson LE, et al. Age-related changes in total and regional fat distribution. Ageing Res Rev 2009;8:339–48.
14. Guilherme A, Virbasius JV, Puri V, et al. Adipocyte dysfunctions linking obesity to insulin resistance and type 2 diabetes. Nat Rev Mol Cell Biol 2008;9:367–77.

15. Evans WJ. Skeletal muscle loss: cachexia, sarcopenia, and inactivity. Am J Clin Nutr 2010;91:1123S–7S.
16. Kim JA, Wei Y, Sowers RJ. Role of mitochondrial dysfunction in insulin resistance. Circ Res 2008;102:401–14.
17. Szoke E, Shrayyef MZ, Messing S, et al. Effect of aging on glucose homeostasis: accelerated deterioration of β-cell function in individuals with impaired glucose tolerance. Diabetes Care 2008;31:539–43.
18. Dehghan A, Kardys I, de Maat MP, et al. Genetic variation, C-reactive protein levels, and incidence of diabetes. Diabetes 2007;56:872–8.
19. Bergman H, Ferrucci L, Guralnik J, et al. Frailty: an emerging research and clinical paradigm-issues and controversies. J Gerontol A Biol Sci Med Sci 2009;62A: 731–7.
20. Fried LP, Tangen CM, Walston J, et al. Frailty in older adults: evidence for a phenotype. J Gerontol A Biol Sci Med Sci 2001;56A:M146–56.
21. Beers MH, Berkow R, editors. The Merck manual of geriatrics. Medical services, USMEDSA, USHH. Section 1. Nutritional disorders. Malnutrition; 2000–2004. Chapter 2. Available at: www.merck.com/mrkshared/mmanual/section/chapter2/2a.jsp. Accessed February 01, 2015.
22. Lee JS, Auyeung TW, Leung J, et al. The effect of diabetes mellitus on age-associated lean mass loss in 3153 older adults. Diabet Med 2010;27:1366–71.
23. Landi F, Onder G, Bernabei R. Sarcopenia and diabetes: two sides of the same coin. J Am Med Dir Assoc 2013;14:540–1.
24. Leenders M, Verdijk LB, van der Hoeven L, et al. Patients with type 2 diabetes show a greater decline in muscle mass, muscle strength, and functional capacity with aging. J Am Med Dir Assoc 2013;14:585–92.
25. Rizvi AA. Nutritional challenges in the elderly with diabetes. Int J Diabetes Mellit 2009;1:26–31.
26. Volpato S, Maraldi C, Fellin R. Type 2 diabetes and risk for functional decline and disability in older persons. Curr Diabetes Rev 2010;6:134–43.
27. Gregg EW, Beckles GL, Williamson DF, et al. Diabetes and physical disability among older U.S. adults. Diabetes Care 2000;23:1272–7.
28. Volpato S, Blaum C, Resnick H, et al. Comorbidities and impairments explaining the association between diabetes and lower extremities disabilities. Diabetes Care 2002;25:678–83.
29. Gregg EW, Mangione CM, Cauley JA, et al, Study of Osteoporotic Fractures Research Group. Diabetes and incidence of functional disability in older women. Diabetes Care 2002;25:61–7.
30. Stewart KJ. Exercise training and the cardiovascular consequences of type 2 diabetes and hypertension: plausible mechanisms for improving cardiovascular health. JAMA 2002;288:1622–31.
31. Knowler WC, Fowler SE, Hamman RF, et al, Diabetes Prevention Program Research Group. 10-year follow-up of diabetes incidence and weight loss in the Diabetes Prevention Program outcomes study. Lancet 2009;374:1677–86.
32. Kumar V, Atherton P, Smith K, et al. Human muscle protein synthesis and breakdown during and after exercise. J Appl Physiol (1985) 2009;106:2026–39.
33. Bauer J, Biolo G, Cederholm T, et al. Evidence-based recommendations for optimal dietary protein intake in older people: a position paper from the PROT-AGE Study Group. J Am Med Dir Assoc 2013;14:542–59.
34. KDOQI. KDOQI clinical practice guidelines and clinical practice recommendations for diabetes and chronic kidney disease. Am J Kidney Dis 2007;49: S12–154.

35. Larsen RN, Mann NJ, Maclean E, et al. The effect of high-protein, low carbohydrate diets in the treatment of type 2 diabetes: a 12 month randomised controlled trial. Diabetologia 2011;54:731–40.
36. Yang Y, Breen L, Burd NA, et al. Resistance exercise enhances myofibrillar protein synthesis with graded intakes of whey protein in older men. Br J Nutr 2012; 108:1780–8.
37. Fujita S, Dreyer HC, Drummond MJ, et al. Nutrient signalling in the regulation of human muscle protein synthesis. J Physiol 2007;582:813–23.
38. Smith GI, Atherton P, Reeds DN, et al. Dietary omega-3 fatty acid supplementation increases the rate of muscle protein synthesis in older adults: a randomized controlled trial. Am J Clin Nutr 2011;93:402–12.
39. Ellis J, Johnson MA, Fischer JG, et al. Nutrition and health education intervention for whole grain foods in the Georgia older Americans nutrition programs. J Nutr Elder 2005;24:67–83.
40. Greenhaff PL, Karagounis LG, Peirce N, et al. Disassociation between the effects of amino acids and insulin on signaling, ubiquitin ligases, and protein turnover in human muscle. Am J Physiol Endocrinol Metab 2008;295:E595–604.
41. Seok WP, Goodpaster BH, Jung SL, et al. Excessive loss of skeletal muscle mass in older adults with type 2 diabetes. Diabetes Care 2009;32:1993–7.
42. Yang Z, Scott CA, Mao C, et al. Resistance exercise versus aerobic exercise for type 2 diabetes: a systematic review and meta-analysis. Sports Med 2014;44:487–99.
43. Brooks N, Layne JE, Gordon PL, et al. Strength training improves muscle quality and insulin sensitivity in Hispanic older adults with type 2 diabetes. Int J Med Sci 2007;4:19–27.
44. Irvine C, Taylor NF. Progressive resistance exercise improves glycaemic control in people with type 2 diabetes mellitus: a systematic review. Aust J Physiother 2009; 55:237–46.
45. Hovanec N, Sawant A, Overend TJ, et al. Resistance training and older adults with type 2 diabetes mellitus: strength of the evidence. J Aging Res 2012; 2012:284635.
46. Davidson LE, Hudson R, Kilpatrick K, et al. Effects of exercise modality on insulin resistance and functional limitation in older adults. A randomized controlled trial. Arch Intern Med 2009;169:122–31.
47. Rennie MJ, Wackerhage H, Spangenburg EE, et al. Control of the size of the human muscle mass. Annu Rev Physiol 2004;66:799–828.
48. Tieland M, Dirks ML, van der Zwaluw N, et al. Protein supplementation increases muscle mass gain during prolonged resistance-type exercise training in frail elderly people: a randomized, double-blind, placebo controlled trial. J Am Med Dir Assoc 2012;13:713–9.
49. Rahi B, Morais JA, Dionne IJ, et al. The combined effects of diet quality and physical activity on maintenance of muscle strength among diabetic older adults from the NuAge cohort. Exp Gerontol 2014;49:40–6.
50. Diabetes Prevention Program Research Group. Reduction in the incidence of type 2 diabetes with lifestyle intervention or metformin. N Engl J Med 2002;346: 393–403.
51. Espeland MA, Rejeski WJ, West DS, et al. Intensive weight loss intervention in older individuals: results from the Action for Health in Diabetes type 2 diabetes mellitus trial. J Am Geriatr Soc 2013;61:912–22.
52. Rejeski WJ, Ip EH, Bertoni AG, et al, Look AHEAD Research Group. Life style change and mobility in obese adults with type 2 diabetes. N Engl J Med 2012; 366:1209–17.

53. Fiatarone M, O'Neill EF, Ryan ND, et al. Exercise training and nutritional supplementation for physical frailty in very elderly people. N Engl J Med 1994;330:1769–75.
54. Valenzuela T. Efficacy of progressive resistance training interventions in older adults in nursing homes: a systematic review. J Am Med Dir Assoc 2012;13:418–28.
55. Sinclair AJ, Task and Finish Group of Diabetes UK. Good clinical practice guidelines for care home residents with diabetes: an executive summary. Diabet Med 2011;28:772–7.

Nutrition and Cognition in Aging Adults

Nicola Coley, PhD[a,b,c,*,1], Charlotte Vaurs, MD[a,b,d,1], Sandrine Andrieu, MD, PhD[a,b,c]

KEYWORDS

- Cognitive decline • Dementia • Nutrients • Antioxidants • Vitamins
- Polyunsaturated fatty acids

KEY POINTS

- Numerous longitudinal observational studies have suggested that nutrients, such as antioxidants, B vitamins, and ω-3 fatty acids, may prevent cognitive decline or dementia.
- There is very little evidence from well-sized randomized controlled trials (RCTs) that nutritional interventions can benefit cognition in later life.
- Nutritional interventions may be more effective in individuals with poorer nutritional status or as part of multidomain interventions simultaneously targeting multiple lifestyle factors.
- Further evidence, notably from RCTs, is required to prove or refute these hypotheses.

INTRODUCTION

The prevalence of dementia, including its most common form, Alzheimer disease (AD), is currently estimated at 36 million people worldwide. Given the expected increase in the number of dementia cases worldwide in the coming years due to demographic aging,[1] finding interventions able to prevent cognitive decline or dementia is a currently a research priority.[2]

Numerous observational studies have suggested a relationship between lifestyle factors, including nutrition and diet, and cognitive function in aging adults (**Table 1**). Some micronutrients, including the B vitamins, antioxidant vitamins, certain essential minerals, and essential fatty acids, as well as macronutrients and dietary patterns, are thought to play a key role in cognitive function, with a large base of evidence from numerous mechanistic animal studies.[3]

Funding Sources: None.
Conflict of Interest: None.

[a] INSERM UMR 1027, 37 allées Jules Guesde, Toulouse F-31073, France; [b] University of Toulouse III, 37 allées Jules Guesde, Toulouse F-31073, France; [c] Department of Epidemiology and Public Health, CHU Toulouse, 37 allées Jules Guesde, Toulouse F-31073, France; [d] Nutrition Unit, Department of Endocrinology, CHU Toulouse, 24 chemin de Pouvourville, Toulouse F-31059, France
[1] Authors contributed equally to this work.
* Corresponding author. Inserm UMR 1027, 37 allées Jules Guesde, Toulouse F-31073, France.
E-mail address: coley.n@chu-toulouse.fr

Clin Geriatr Med 31 (2015) 453–464
http://dx.doi.org/10.1016/j.cger.2015.04.008 geriatric.theclinics.com

Table 1
Types of studies used to evaluate the effect of nutrition on cognition

	Physiopathology	Prospective Observational Studies	Systematic Review/ Meta-Analysis of Prospective Observational Studies	RCTs	Systematic Review/Meta-Analysis of RCTs
Antioxidants	X	X	X	X	—
Polyphenols	X	X	—	X	—
PUFA	X	X	X	X	X
B Vitamins	X	X	X	X	X
Vitamin D	X	X	X	—	—
Calorie restriction	X	—	X	—	—
MeDi	X	X	X	X	—

The aim of this article is to give an update on the current knowledge regarding the role of nutrition in the prevention of cognitive decline or dementia, based on the results of prospective studies, in particular, randomized controlled trials (RCTs), and to highlight future research perspectives.

SUMMARY OF FINDINGS

The findings from prospective observational studies and RCTs are described below, and the types of studies conducted for each type of nutrient or dietary pattern are summarized in **Table 1**.

Antioxidants

Because the brain is an organ with a high metabolic rate, oxidative stress, which may influence neurodegeneration and neuronal death in AD,[4] is a common phenomenon in its neural tissues.[5] Exogenous antioxidants, including vitamins A (eg, β-carotene), C, and E (tocopherols), and trace minerals, such as manganese, copper, selenium, and zinc, may protect against oxidative stress and could prevent cognitive decline or dementia.

Prospective observational studies

A meta-analysis of 7 cohort studies suggested that higher dietary intakes of vitamins E and C were significantly associated with a decreased risk of AD.[6] The association between β-carotene and risk of dementia was borderline significant. However, a more recent systematic review of 10 population-based cohort studies, which took into account methodological quality, found only limited evidence of a possible protective role of antioxidants on cognitive decline in older adults.[7] This review included biological measures of nutrient status or dietary intakes, and heterogeneous results meant that it was not possible to identify a specific antioxidant nutrient that could be recommended or would merit further study.

Randomized controlled trials

No systematic reviews or meta-analyses of RCTs testing antioxidants in a preventive setting were identified. One trial conducted in individuals with mild cognitive impairment (MCI) found no effect of vitamin E on conversion to AD-dementia after 3 years.[8] In cognitively healthy populations, the cognitive effects of antioxidants have mainly been tested in add-on studies in trials initially designed for other purposes, and no beneficial effect was observed.[9–11] Of 4 RCTs that measured cognitive performance at one time point only, in one case several years after the end of antioxidant supplementation,[12] 2 studies found no effect of supplements containing vitamin E, vitamin C, and β-carotene on cognitive performance or dementia,[13,14] and 2 studies found significant beneficial effects.[12,15] One ongoing trial is testing the efficacy of vitamin E and selenium versus placebo on the incidence of AD in an ancillary study to a cancer prevention trial, but conclusions from this large trial may be limited by lower than expected statistical power, because of the effect of enrolling a too healthy cohort, and shortened treatment duration.[16]

Summary

There is little evidence of a protective effect of antioxidants on cognition. However, there have been relatively few trials specifically designed to test this hypothesis, in particular in individuals without cognitive impairment. Furthermore, based on subgroup analyses of the Women's Health Study,[9] some investigators have suggested that vitamin E supplementation may only be beneficial for cognition in individuals with dietary intakes of vitamin E well below the recommended daily allowance.[17] In addition, the cognitive effects of vitamin E may differ by tocopherol subtype.[18] Further well-designed RCTs of antioxidants may therefore be merited, although it should be noted that observational evidence comes primarily from studies that have assessed antioxidants via food frequency questionnaires, which are prone to recall and measurement bias, and furthermore, the potential harmful effects of high-dose vitamin E must not be ignored.[19]

Polyphenols

Like antioxidant vitamins, dietary polyphenols, one of the most abundant antioxidants in the human diet, can contribute to the regulation of oxidative stress.[20] They also play a role in regulating vascular health.[21,22] Anti-inflammatory mechanisms probably mediate part of this action.[21] Evidence from in vitro and in vivo studies of polyphenols have demonstrated that they may play an integral role in preventing and treating diseases associated with neurodegeneration due to oxidative stress.[23–26]

Prospective observational studies

A systematic review studying the impact of alcohol on AD indicated that alcohol should not be recommended as a means to decrease risk of developing AD, based on evidence from almost 20 studies.[27] Other studies involving more than 2000 participants have found a beneficial effect of tea consumption on cognitive impairment after 1 to 2 years of follow-up,[28] and a positive association between total polyphenol intake and cognitive factors reflecting language and verbal memory, after a follow-up of 13 years.[29]

Randomized controlled trials

Of 3 short ($\leq$2 months) trials of cocoa flavanols in up to 100 middle-aged or older individuals with normal cognition or MCI, one found beneficial effects of high-dose and intermediate-dose supplementation, compared with low-dose supplementation, on measures of executive function but not on Mini-Mental Status Examination score,[30] and the other 2 found no beneficial effects.[31,32] Other trials, whose small sizes preclude drawing any meaningful conclusions, have tested the cognitive effects of Concord grape juice,[33,34] and Pinus radiata bark extract.[35]

Summary

Most studies on polyphenols have been conducted with animal models and may not be easily generalized to humans. There is not enough research to draw conclusions from observational or randomized studies in humans. Future research should seek to understand how diets rich in polyphenols work in combination with other lifestyle factors to provide neuroprotective properties.

Polyunsaturated Fatty Acids

Polyunsaturated fatty acids (PUFA) are an important component of neural membrane phospholipids and could be involved in the maintenance of cognitive function or prevention of dementia by maintaining membrane integrity and neuronal function or via their antithrombotic and anti-inflammatory properties.[36,37]

Prospective observational studies

A systematic review identified 8 cohort studies that examined the effects of dietary intake of fish or general PUFA or serum concentrations of PUFA on dementia and AD incidence. Two of the studies reported a reduced risk of dementia or AD with increased fish, total ω-3 PUFA, or docosahexaenoic acid (DHA) consumption, while the others found no significant effects.[38] A second review noted that 3 studies that measured cognitive decline all reported significant benefits, although in 2 studies exposure was based on dietary histories.[39]

Randomized controlled trials

A recent *Cochrane Review* identified 3 RCTs of ω-3 PUFA for the prevention of cognitive decline. These trials included 4080 cognitively healthy participants with between 6 and 40 months of follow-up, but no benefit of ω-3 was observed.[40]

Additional trials include a 6-month trial of DHA in 485 individuals aged 55 and older with age-related cognitive decline that found significant beneficial effects on cognitive performance on one coprimary outcome measure only[41]; 2 very small (N <55) trials of 4 to 6 months' duration of eicosapentaenoic acid, DHA, lutein, or DHA and lutein supplementation,[42,43] one of which provided exploratory evidence of short-term beneficial cognitive effects[42]; and an ancillary study of a secondary prevention trial for cardiovascular disease involving 439 individuals that found no significant effects of ω-3 PUFA on cognitive performance measured after 4 years of follow-up.[44]

Summary

Currently, there is very little evidence of a protective role of PUFA on cognitive decline or dementia from RCTs, and results of observational studies should be interpreted with caution.[45] Results of well-sized ongoing RCTs should be examined.[46–48] Previous methodological limitations that would merit particular consideration in new trials include relatively short durations of supplementation and limited cognitive decline in both intervention and control groups during follow-up.[40]

B Vitamins

Increased serum homocysteine is both neurotoxic and a vascular risk factor and has been associated with the development of AD and cognitive impairment in animal models.[49] Homocysteine levels increase when folate and vitamin B12 are deficient, which may contribute to amyloid and tau protein accumulation and neuronal death.[33]

Prospective observational studies

Increased levels of homocysteine have consistently been found to be significantly associated with the risk of cognitive decline or dementia/AD in meta-analyses of cohort studies.[50–52] However, systematic reviews of studies examining the relationship between vitamin B12 and cognitive decline or dementia were inconclusive, although it was noted that the few studies using more sensitive markers of vitamin

B12 status (methylmalonic acid and holotranscobalamin) found the most consistent results.[53,54]

Randomized controlled trials

A systematic review concluded that there was insufficient evidence to draw definitive conclusions about the efficacy of B vitamins (B6, B12, and folate) for cognitive decline or dementia prevention,[38] whereas a more recent meta-analysis of 19 RCTs concluded that B-vitamin supplementation did not improve cognitive function.[55]

Two trials have evaluated the effects of 2-year supplementation with B vitamins on biomarkers: one found a significantly decreased annual rate of brain atrophy compared with placebo in 187 individuals with MCI,[56] but no effect on cognitive function in the total population,[57] and a second trial found a borderline significant ($P = .08$) reduction in plasma Aβ40 levels, compared with placebo in 299 older men.[58]

Summary

Although supplementation with B vitamins did lower homocysteine in the RCTs, there is no conclusive evidence of protection against cognitive decline or dementia. It has been suggested that targeting individuals with raised homocysteine levels may be necessary for efficacy,[59] which is supported by the results of 2 trials,[57,60] but not by a third.[61] The dose or timing of B-vitamin supplementation may also be important.[62]

Vitamin D

Vitamin D may affect cognition through various pathways, including anti-inflammatory and antioxidant effects, and regulation of the genetic expression of neurotrophins and neurotransmitters.[63,64]

Prospective observational studies

A recent systematic review[64] identified 6 prospective studies that measured serum 25OHD concentrations, of which 4 observed a statistically significant decline on cognitive function or a higher incidence of dementia in participants with lower vitamin D levels (after 4–7 years of follow-up).

Summary

Prospective observational studies generally support the hypothesis that lower serum vitamin D levels are associated with cognitive decline in late life, but no completed trials of vitamin D were identified. However, several trials are ongoing, including 2 relatively large-scale RCTs, which are testing vitamin D alone and in combination with ω-3 PUFA and exercise in cognitively normal older adults (clinicaltrials.gov identifiers: NCT01669915 and NCT01745263).

Dietary Patterns

Three biological mechanisms, which are the impact on the vascular system, the impact on oxidative stress, and the attenuation of inflammatory pathway, have been proposed to support that diet, in particular the Mediterranean diet (MeDi), could reduce the risk of dementia.

Even though various dietary patterns have been studied (eg, Japanese diet,[65] and fruit and vegetable consumption[66]), the MeDi has received the most attention.

Mediterranean diet

An increasing body of evidence has supported the role of the MeDi in protecting cognition. The MeDi is characterized by a high intake of fruits, vegetables, cereals, fish, and monounsaturated fatty acids (MUFA). The MeDi is suggested to have the potential to protect against age-related cognitive decline and cognitive impairment. Extra virgin olive oil (EVOO) is not only rich in MUFA but also rich in polyphenols, with a proven anti-inflammatory and antioxidant action, which alone could explain the beneficial impact of EVOO consumption on the brain.[67,68]

Prospective observational studies In a recent systematic review, higher adherence to MeDi was associated with better cognitive function, lower rates of cognitive decline, and reduced risk of AD in 9 of 12 eligible studies, whereas results for MCI were inconsistent.[69]

Randomized controlled trials A large RCT study of long-term supplementation with EVOO—a good source of MUFA—showed significant improvement in verbal fluency and episodic memory, and reduced incidence of MCI, in the supplemented group as compared with controls.[70]

Another RCT in old-age hostel residents showed that regular group dietary counseling and menu changes (based around MeDi) did not lead to a significant reduction in cognitive decline or dementia.[71] There was, however, a borderline trend of less cognitive decline in the cognitively normal at month 24.

Another large RCT of dietary patterns and health based on the MeDi approach is ongoing. New dietary strategies addressing the specific needs of the elderly population for healthy aging in Europe (NU-AGE) is a European multicenter study focused on older adults and includes in-depth cognitive assessments.[72]

Summary Available evidence suggests that the MeDi might exert a long-term beneficial effect on brain functioning. More high-powered observational studies with long-term follow-up for cognition and RCTs assessing the impact of shifting to a MeDi on cognitive functions are still needed.[73]

Calorie restriction

Dietary energy restriction enhances neural plasticity and reduces vulnerability of the brain.[74] Calorie restriction may have a protective effect on the cognitive decline via up-regulation of brain-derived neurotrophic factor and reduction of the oxidative stress in the hippocampus.[75]

Randomized controlled trials A first RCT showed that calorie restriction was not associated with a consistent pattern of cognitive impairment.[76] However, this RCT had limitations (small sample size, limited statistical power), whereas another RCT found a favorable effect of an energy-restricted low-fat diet compared with an isocaloric low-carbohydrate diet on mood state and affect in overweight and obese individuals.[77] Working memory and speed of processing were not affected by the low-fat diet.

Summary Even though calorie restriction seems to protect against cognitive decline in animal models, there is no conclusive evidence of protection against cognitive decline or dementia in RCTs.

DISCUSSION

Although many observational studies have provided evidence of a protective role of nutrition against cognitive decline or dementia onset, no randomized trial has conclusively demonstrated efficacy of a nutritional intervention.

A first explanation for these differing results is the methodology of the observational studies that are more susceptible to bias and confounding than RCTs. Measurement (or recall) bias is a particular concern in studies assessing the role of nutritional factors in the prevention of dementia or cognitive decline, because intakes are often quantified based on self-reported questionnaires only. Furthermore, there may be seasonal variations in the diet and nutritional intake of the subjects under study that may not be taken into account if exposure is measured at one time point. Confounding is also a major risk factor in observational studies. In the case of studies on nutrition and cognitive decline/dementia risk, nutritional status could also be an indicator of previous life experiences,[78] such as education level or socioeconomic status. Most longitudinal studies adjust for subjects' level of education in their analyses, but other indicators of socioeconomic status are less often considered. Nutritional status could also indicate a healthy lifestyle in general, and so the seemingly protective role of nutrition may actually reflect a protective effect of an overall healthy lifestyle.

Second, methodological differences between RCTs and observational studies should be considered.[79,80] When nutritional status is measured in observational studies, it is likely to be a reflection of long-term exposure, and dietary intakes in previous times throughout the life course could have more of an impact than current intake. In RCTs, however, nutritional interventions are usually given for relatively short periods, meaning that the intervention may not be tested at the right time or for long enough period of time.

Also, RCTs may not be recruiting or even targeting the individuals in most need of intervention. Prevention trials in general tend to include participants who are more highly educated and healthier than the general population,[81,82] and probably also therefore have better nutritional status. Supplementation with certain nutrients, in particular vitamins B or E, may only be effective in individuals with poor nutritional status, but only a few RCTs were designed to test this hypothesis.[17,59] Furthermore, the neurodegenerative process of dementia begins long before any clinical signs become apparent, and nutrients may affect this process at an early stage.[83] Interventions carried out later in life may have less effect than if they were carried out at a younger age, although most observational studies also focused on older populations.

The doses of nutrients used in supplements in RCTs may also be important, with the highest doses not necessarily being optimal.[62]

It is interesting to note that one of the few trials of B vitamins that was able to demonstrate a beneficial effect on cognition used a moderate dose of B vitamins in a target population that was aged 50 to 70 years and had a suboptimal nutritional status.[60]

Heterogeneity in outcome measures must also be considered. Nutrient intakes were found to be related to dementia incidence in some longitudinal studies, but none of the RCTs testing nutritional interventions have measured dementia incidence as an outcome. The clinical relevance of small beneficial effects on measures of cognitive decline must be considered, and such results should be put into context, for example, by comparing intervention effects to the effects of other factors, such as age.[60] Moreover, it is important to note that the available RCTs have used a plethora of different cognitive tests to study the effects of nutritional interventions, thereby making it difficult for comparison among studies and for overall data interpretation.

The association between nutrition and cognition is complex, and it is unlikely that one nutrient alone will play a major role. From a public health perspective, it is now important to research in more depth the associations between groups of nutrients or particular dietary habits that may have an impact on cognition. Furthermore, nutritional interventions may have synergistic effects with other lifestyle interventions (eg, physical exercise, social interactions, mental stimulation),[84] highlighting the importance of "multidomain" RCTs testing interventions targeting multiple risk or protective factors simultaneously. The results of the first large multidomain trials are eagerly awaited.[48,85]

SUMMARY

RCTs have so far mainly tested supplements targeting a specific type of nutrient and have provided very little evidence that nutritional interventions can benefit cognition in later life. Specific dietary patterns, like the MeDi, may be more beneficial than a high consumption of individual nutrients, and research has recently started to focus on this. There is a need for well-designed, large-scale, long-term RCTs in healthy adults, in particular to test the effects of targeted supplementation in individuals with poor nutritional status. Interventions based around dietary patterns could also be tested; however, more high-powered observational studies with long-term follow-up for cognition and RCTs assessing the impact of shifting to a MeDi on cognitive functions are still needed in various populations.[73]

REFERENCES

1. Prince M, Bryce R, Albanese E, et al. The global prevalence of dementia: a systematic review and metaanalysis. Alzheimers Dement 2013;9:63–75.e2.
2. Prince M, Albanese E, Guerchet M, et al. World Alzheimer report 2014 dementia and risk reduction: an analysis of protective and modifiable factors. London: Alzheimer's Disease International; 2014.
3. Joseph J, Cole G, Head E, et al. Nutrition, brain aging, and neurodegeneration. J Neurosci 2009;29:12795–801.
4. Markesbery WR, Carney JM. Oxidative alterations in Alzheimer's disease. Brain Pathol 1999;9:133–46.
5. Bishop NA, Lu T, Yankner BA. Neural mechanisms of ageing and cognitive decline. Nature 2010;464:529–35.
6. Li FJ, Shen L, Ji HF. Dietary intakes of vitamin E, vitamin C, and beta-carotene and risk of Alzheimer's disease: a meta-analysis. J Alzheimers Dis 2012;31:253–8.
7. Rafnsson SB, Dilis V, Trichopoulou A. Antioxidant nutrients and age-related cognitive decline: a systematic review of population-based cohort studies. Eur J Nutr 2013;52:1553–67.
8. Petersen RC, Thomas RG, Grundman M, et al. Vitamin E and donepezil for the treatment of mild cognitive impairment. N Engl J Med 2005;352:2379–88.
9. Kang JH, Cook N, Manson J, et al. A randomized trial of vitamin E supplementation and cognitive function in women. Arch Intern Med 2006;166:2462–8.
10. Kang JH, Cook NR, Manson JE, et al. Vitamin E, vitamin C, beta carotene, and cognitive function among women with or at risk of cardiovascular disease: the women's antioxidant and cardiovascular study. Circulation 2009;119:2772–80.
11. Smith A, Clarke R, Nutt D, et al. Anti-oxidant vitamins and mental performance of the elderly. Hum Psychopharmacol 1999;14:459–71.
12. Kesse-Guyot E, Fezeu L, Jeandel C, et al. French adults' cognitive performance after daily supplementation with antioxidant vitamins and minerals at nutritional doses: a post hoc analysis of the Supplementation in Vitamins and Mineral Antioxidants (SU.VI.MAX) trial. Am J Clin Nutr 2011;94:892–9.
13. MRC/BHF Heart Protection Study of antioxidant vitamin supplementation in 20,536 high-risk individuals: a randomised placebo-controlled trial. Lancet 2002;360:23–33.

14. Yaffe K, Clemons TE, McBee WL, et al. Impact of antioxidants, zinc, and copper on cognition in the elderly: a randomized, controlled trial. Neurology 2004;63: 1705–7.
15. Grodstein F, Kang JH, Glynn RJ, et al. A randomized trial of beta carotene supplementation and cognitive function in men: the Physicians' Health Study II. Arch Intern Med 2007;167:2184–90.
16. Kryscio RJ, Abner EL, Schmitt FA, et al. A randomized controlled Alzheimer's disease prevention trial's evolution into an exposure trial: the PREADViSE Trial. J Nutr Health Aging 2013;17:72–5.
17. Barnes JL, Tian M, Edens NK, et al. Consideration of nutrient levels in studies of cognitive decline. Nutr Rev 2014;72:707–19.
18. Morris MC, Evans DA, Tangney CC, et al. Relation of the tocopherol forms to incident Alzheimer disease and to cognitive change. Am J Clin Nutr 2005;81:508–14.
19. Bjelakovic G, Nikolova D, Gluud LL, et al. Mortality in randomized trials of antioxidant supplements for primary and secondary prevention: systematic review and meta-analysis. JAMA 2007;297:842–57.
20. Stevenson DE, Hurst RD. Polyphenolic phytochemicals–just antioxidants or much more? Cell Mol Life Sci 2007;64:2900–16.
21. Cherniack EP. A berry thought-provoking idea: the potential role of plant polyphenols in the treatment of age-related cognitive disorders. Br J Nutr 2012;108: 794–800.
22. Ghosh D, Scheepens A. Vascular action of polyphenols. Mol Nutr Food Res 2009; 53:322–31.
23. Scalbert A, Johnson IT, Saltmarsh M. Polyphenols: antioxidants and beyond. Am J Clin Nutr 2005;81:215S–7S.
24. Davinelli S, Sapere N, Zella D, et al. Pleiotropic protective effects of phytochemicals in Alzheimer's disease. Oxid Med Cell Longev 2012;2012:386527.
25. Ho L, Chen LH, Wang J, et al. Heterogeneity in red wine polyphenolic contents differentially influences Alzheimer's disease-type neuropathology and cognitive deterioration. J Alzheimers Dis 2009;16:59–72.
26. Wang J, Ferruzzi MG, Ho L, et al. Brain-targeted proanthocyanidin metabolites for Alzheimer's disease treatment. J Neurosci 2012;32:5144–50.
27. Piazza-Gardner AK, Gaffud TJ, Barry AE. The impact of alcohol on Alzheimer's disease: a systematic review. Aging Ment Health 2013;17:133–46.
28. Ng TP, Feng L, Niti M, et al. Tea consumption and cognitive impairment and decline in older Chinese adults. Am J Clin Nutr 2008;88:224–31.
29. Kesse-Guyot E, Fezeu L, Andreeva VA, et al. Total and specific polyphenol intakes in midlife are associated with cognitive function measured 13 years later. J Nutr 2012;142:76–83.
30. Desideri G, Kwik-Uribe C, Grassi D, et al. Benefits in cognitive function, blood pressure, and insulin resistance through cocoa flavanol consumption in elderly subjects with mild cognitive impairment: the Cocoa, Cognition, and Aging (CoCoA) study. Hypertension 2012;60:794–801.
31. Camfield DA, Scholey A, Pipingas A, et al. Steady state visually evoked potential (SSVEP) topography changes associated with cocoa flavanol consumption. Physiol Behav 2012;105:948–57.
32. Crews WD Jr, Harrison DW, Wright JW. A double-blind, placebo-controlled, randomized trial of the effects of dark chocolate and cocoa on variables associated with neuropsychological functioning and cardiovascular health: clinical findings from a sample of healthy, cognitively intact older adults. Am J Clin Nutr 2008; 87:872–80.

33. Krikorian R, Nash TA, Shidler MD, et al. Concord grape juice supplementation improves memory function in older adults with mild cognitive impairment. Br J Nutr 2010;103:730–4.
34. Krikorian R, Boespflug EL, Fleck DE, et al. Concord grape juice supplementation and neurocognitive function in human aging. J Agric Food Chem 2012;60: 5736–42.
35. Pipingas A, Silberstein RB, Vitetta L, et al. Improved cognitive performance after dietary supplementation with a Pinus radiata bark extract formulation. Phytother Res 2008;22:1168–74.
36. Uauy R, Dangour AD. Nutrition in brain development and aging: role of essential fatty acids. Nutr Rev 2006;64:S24–33 [discussion: S72–91].
37. Gillette-Guyonnet S, Secher M, Vellas B. Nutrition and neurodegeneration: epidemiological evidence and challenges for future research. Br J Clin Pharmacol 2013;75:738–55.
38. Dangour AD, Whitehouse PJ, Rafferty K, et al. B-vitamins and fatty acids in the prevention and treatment of Alzheimer's disease and dementia: a systematic review. J Alzheimers Dis 2010;22:205–24.
39. Fotuhi M, Mohassel P, Yaffe K. Fish consumption, long-chain omega-3 fatty acids and risk of cognitive decline or Alzheimer disease: a complex association. Nat Clin Pract Neurol 2009;5:140–52.
40. Sydenham E, Dangour AD, Lim WS. Omega 3 fatty acid for the prevention of cognitive decline and dementia. Cochrane Database Syst Rev 2012;(6):CD005379.
41. Yurko-Mauro K, McCarthy D, Rom D, et al. Beneficial effects of docosahexaenoic acid on cognition in age-related cognitive decline. Alzheimers Dement 2010;6: 456–64.
42. Johnson EJ, McDonald K, Caldarella SM, et al. Cognitive findings of an exploratory trial of docosahexaenoic acid and lutein supplementation in older women. Nutr Neurosci 2008;11:75–83.
43. Sinn N, Milte CM, Street SJ, et al. Effects of n-3 fatty acids, EPA v. DHA, on depressive symptoms, quality of life, memory and executive function in older adults with mild cognitive impairment: a 6-month randomised controlled trial. Br J Nutr 2012;107:1682–93.
44. Andreeva VA, Kesse-Guyot E, Barberger-Gateau P, et al. Cognitive function after supplementation with B vitamins and long-chain omega-3 fatty acids: ancillary findings from the SU.FOL.OM3 randomized trial. Am J Clin Nutr 2011;94: 278–86.
45. Williams J, Plassman B, Burke J, et al. Preventing Alzheimer's disease and cognitive decline. Evidence report/technology assessment no. 193. (Prepared by the Duke Evidence-Based Practice Center under contract no. HHSA 290-2007-10066-I.) AHRQ publication no. 10-E005. Rockville (MD): Agency for Healthcare Research and Quality; 2010.
46. Danthiir V, Burns NR, Nettelbeck T, et al. The older people, omega-3, and cognitive health (EPOCH) trial design and methodology: a randomised, double-blind, controlled trial investigating the effect of long-chain omega-3 fatty acids on cognitive ageing and wellbeing in cognitively healthy older adults. Nutr J 2011; 10:117.
47. Manson JE, Bassuk SS, Lee IM, et al. The VITamin D and OmegA-3 TriaL (VITAL): rationale and design of a large randomized controlled trial of vitamin D and marine omega-3 fatty acid supplements for the primary prevention of cancer and cardiovascular disease. Contemp Clin Trials 2012;33:159–71.

48. Vellas B, Carrie I, Gillette-Guyonnet S, et al. MAPT study: a multidomain approach for preventing Alzheimer's disease: design and baseline data. J Prev Alzheimers Disease 2014;1:13–22.
49. Kruman II, Kumaravel TS, Lohani A, et al. Folic acid deficiency and homocysteine impair DNA repair in hippocampal neurons and sensitize them to amyloid toxicity in experimental models of Alzheimer's disease. J Neurosci 2002;22:1752–62.
50. Nie T, Lu T, Xie L, et al. Hyperhomocysteinemia and risk of cognitive decline: a meta-analysis of prospective cohort studies. Eur Neurol 2014;72:241–8.
51. Wald DS, Kasturiratne A, Simmonds M. Serum homocysteine and dementia: meta-analysis of eight cohort studies including 8669 participants. Alzheimers Dement 2011;7:412–7.
52. Beydoun MA, Beydoun HA, Gamaldo AA, et al. Epidemiologic studies of modifiable factors associated with cognition and dementia: systematic review and meta-analysis. BMC Public Health 2014;14:643.
53. Doets EL, van Wijngaarden JP, Szczecinska A, et al. Vitamin B12 intake and status and cognitive function in elderly people. Epidemiol Rev 2013;35:2–21.
54. O'Leary F, Allman-Farinelli M, Samman S. Vitamin B_{12} status, cognitive decline and dementia: a systematic review of prospective cohort studies. Br J Nutr 2012;108:1948–61.
55. Ford AH, Almeida OP. Effect of homocysteine lowering treatment on cognitive function: a systematic review and meta-analysis of randomized controlled trials. J Alzheimers Dis 2012;29:133–49.
56. Smith AD, Smith SM, de Jager CA, et al. Homocysteine-lowering by B vitamins slows the rate of accelerated brain atrophy in mild cognitive impairment: a randomized controlled trial. PLoS One 2010;5:e12244.
57. de Jager CA, Oulhaj A, Jacoby R, et al. Cognitive and clinical outcomes of homocysteine-lowering B-vitamin treatment in mild cognitive impairment: a randomized controlled trial. Int J Geriatr Psychiatry 2012;27:592–600.
58. Flicker L, Martins RN, Thomas J, et al. B-vitamins reduce plasma levels of beta amyloid. Neurobiol Aging 2008;29:303–5.
59. Morris MC, Tangney CC. A potential design flaw of randomized trials of vitamin supplements. JAMA 2011;305:1348–9.
60. Durga J, van Boxtel MP, Schouten EG, et al. Effect of 3-year folic acid supplementation on cognitive function in older adults in the FACIT trial: a randomised, double blind, controlled trial. Lancet 2007;369:208–16.
61. McMahon JA, Green TJ, Skeaff CM, et al. A controlled trial of homocysteine lowering and cognitive performance. N Engl J Med 2006;354:2764–72.
62. Otaegui-Arrazola A, Amiano P, Elbusto A, et al. Diet, cognition, and Alzheimer's disease: food for thought. Eur J Nutr 2014;53:1–23.
63. McCann JC, Ames BN. Is there convincing biological or behavioral evidence linking vitamin D deficiency to brain dysfunction? FASEB J 2008;22:982–1001.
64. Annweiler C, Montero-Odasso M, Llewellyn DJ, et al. Meta-analysis of memory and executive dysfunctions in relation to vitamin D. J Alzheimers Dis 2013;37:147–71.
65. Ozawa M, Ninomiya T, Ohara T, et al. Dietary patterns and risk of dementia in an elderly Japanese population: the Hisayama Study. Am J Clin Nutr 2013;97:1076–82.
66. Barberger-Gateau P, Raffaitin C, Letenneur L, et al. Dietary patterns and risk of dementia: the Three-City cohort study. Neurology 2007;69:1921–30.
67. Bullo M, Lamuela-Raventos R, Salas-Salvado J. Mediterranean diet and oxidation: nuts and olive oil as important sources of fat and antioxidants. Curr Top Med Chem 2011;11:1797–810.

68. Cicerale S, Lucas LJ, Keast RS. Antimicrobial, antioxidant and anti-inflammatory phenolic activities in extra virgin olive oil. Curr Opin Biotechnol 2012;23:129–35.
69. Lourida I, Soni M, Thompson-Coon J, et al. Mediterranean diet, cognitive function, and dementia: a systematic review. Epidemiology 2013;24:479–89.
70. Martinez-Lapiscina EH, Clavero P, Toledo E, et al. Virgin olive oil supplementation and long-term cognition: the PREDIMED-NAVARRA randomized, trial. J Nutr Health Aging 2013;17:544–52.
71. Kwok TC, Lam LC, Sea MM, et al. A randomized controlled trial of dietetic interventions to prevent cognitive decline in old age hostel residents. Eur J Clin Nutr 2012;66:1135–40.
72. Santoro A, Pini E, Scurti M, et al. Combating inflammaging through a Mediterranean whole diet approach: the NU-AGE project's conceptual framework and design. Mech Ageing Dev 2014;136-137:3–13.
73. Feart C, Samieri C, Barberger-Gateau P. Mediterranean diet and cognitive health: an update of available knowledge. Curr Opin Clin Nutr Metab Care 2015;18:51–62.
74. Mattson MP. The impact of dietary energy intake on cognitive aging. Front Aging Neurosci 2010;2:5.
75. Kishi T, Hirooka Y, Nagayama T, et al. Calorie restriction improves cognitive decline via up-regulation of brain-derived neurotrophic factor. Int Heart J 2014;56:110–5.
76. Martin CK, Anton SD, Han H, et al. Examination of cognitive function during six months of calorie restriction: results of a randomized controlled trial. Rejuvenation Res 2007;10:179–90.
77. Brinkworth GD, Buckley JD, Noakes M, et al. Long-term effects of a very low-carbohydrate diet and a low-fat diet on mood and cognitive function. Arch Intern Med 2009;169:1873–80.
78. Gold D, Andres D, Etezadi J, et al. Structural equation model of intellectual change and continuity and predictors of intelligence in older men. Psychol Aging 1995;10:294–303.
79. Coley N, Andrieu S, Gardette V, et al. Dementia prevention: methodological explanations for inconsistent results. Epidemiol Rev 2008;30:35–66.
80. Caracciolo B, Xu W, Collins S, et al. Cognitive decline, dietary factors and gut-brain interactions. Mech Ageing Dev 2014;136-137:59–69.
81. Green RC, Dekosky ST. Primary prevention trials in Alzheimer disease. Neurology 2006;67:S2–5.
82. Dangour AD, Allen E, Richards M, et al. Design considerations in long-term intervention studies for the prevention of cognitive decline or dementia. Nutr Rev 2010;68(Suppl 1):S16–21.
83. Luchsinger JA, Mayeux R. Dietary factors and Alzheimer's disease. Lancet Neurol 2004;3:579–87.
84. Scarmeas N, Luchsinger JA, Schupf N, et al. Physical activity, diet, and risk of Alzheimer disease. JAMA 2009;302:627–37.
85. Kivipelto M, Solomon A, Ahtiluoto S, et al. The Finnish Geriatric Intervention Study to Prevent Cognitive Impairment and Disability (FINGER): study design and progress. Alzheimers Dement 2013;9:657–65.

Index

Note: Page numbers of article titles are in **boldface** type.

A

Adults, aging, nutrition and cognition in, **453–464**
Alzheimer disease, 404–406, 453
Amino acids, and protein, supplementation with, 331–333
Anorexia, od aging, taste and smell and, 419–420
  of aging, **417–427**
    altered satiety and satiation in, 421
    central hormones and, 422
    cytokines and, 420–421
    loss of appetite in, 418
    loss of muscle mass and strength in, 418
    management of, to achieve healthy aging, 423–425
    neuroendocrine mechanisms and, 421–423
    pathophysiology of, 419
    physiologic factors contributing to, 420
    prevalence of, 418–419
    screening in, 419
  SNAQ screening test for, 436–437
Antioxidants, cognitive decline and, 454–455
Atherosclerosis, 404
  risk of, aging and, 405

B

ß-Carotene, vitamin A and, 356–358
    bone health and, 352
    cancer prevention and, 357–358
    cataracts/macular degeneration and, 358
B vitamins, cognitive function and, 456–457
Blood pressure, gastric emptying and, 347–350
Body mass index, and age, lifestyle recommendations for, 313
  optimizing of, therapeutic options for, 312–313
Body weight, excessive, in older adults, **311–326**
Bone mineral density, protein intake and, 334
Breath tests, to evaluate gastric emptying, 344

C

Calorie restriction, protective effect of, on cognitive decline, 458
Cancer, and vitamin D, 361
  folic acid and, 361
Cancer prevention, vitamin E and, 358

Clin Geriatr Med 31 (2015) 465–470
http://dx.doi.org/10.1016/S0749-0690(15)00046-4 geriatric.theclinics.com

Cardiovascular disease, folic acid and, 361
vitamin D and, 361
vitamin E and, 359
Cardiovascular health, supplements beneficial to, 411
Cataracts, vitamin C and, 359
Cholesterol, aging and, 404
pathological conditions associated with, 404–406
and aging, role of nutrition and physical activity in, **401–416**
nonpharmacologic interventions to control, 413
physical activity/exercise and aging, 411–412
role in body, 403
synthesis, aging and, 403
Cognition, and nutrition, in aging adults, **453–464**
effect of nutrition on, 454
Cognitive decline, antioxidants and, 454–455
Common cold, vitamin C and, 359–360

D

Dehydration, clinical diagnosis of, 390–391
definition of, 390
diagnosis of, algorithmic approach to, 391, 392
fluid replacement in, 392
hypernatremia, and hyponatremia, **389–399**
indicators of, 390
Dementia, risk of, dietary patterns and, 457–458
vitamin E and, 359
Diabetes, and aging, mobility decline in, 442
and frailty of aging, 442
as phenotype in old age, 441–442
effects of aging in, 440–441, 446
epidemiology of, 440
exercise and, 444–445
frailty and, 447
in old age, 439
lifestyle modifications in, 442–445
nutrition, and exercise, **439–451**
nutritional therapy in, 443–444
vitamin D and, 361
Dietary patterns, risk of dementia and, 457–458

E

Exercise, aerobic and resistance, comparison and, 444–445
diabetes and, 444–445
frailty and, 380
nutrition, and diabetes, **439–451**

F

Falls, vitamin D and, 360
Fatty acids, polyunsaturated, cognitive function and, 456

Folic acid, cancer and, 361
cardiovascular disease and, 361
Fractures, associated with hyponatremia, 393
Frailty, as transitional state, 375–376, 377
diabetes and, 447
dynamics of, 377
electrolyte abnormalities in, 389–390
exercise and nutrition, **375–387**
interventions in, 376
combining exercise and nutrition, 380–381
multifactorial randomized controlled, 381–383
key roles in process, messages in, 383–384
nutrition in, 380
of aging, diabetes and, 442
physical, as geriatric syndrome, 369
sarcopenia as biological substrate of, **367–373**
physical exercise in, 379–380
transitions in, factors associated with, 378–379
vulnerability to stressors and, 375

G

Gastric emptying, absorption of medications, energy intake, glycemic control, and blood pressure, 347–350
and motility, effects of healthy aging on, 345–346
control of, intrinsic and extrinsic signals for, 343
delayed, causes of, 347
in elderly, **339–353**
measurement of, 343–345
mechanisms controlling, 340
medical conditions and medications associated with, 346–347
migrating motor complex and, 340–341
motor activity of stomach and, 341
rates and patterns of, 341–342
techniques to evaluate, 343–345
Glycemia, postprandial, determinants of, 348
Glycemic control, gastric emptying and, 347–350

H

Hip fracture, in malnutrition, 333–334
Hypercholesterolemia, caloric restriction in, 406
cholesterol, diet, and aging, 406
dietary fat and, 406
fatty acids and, 406–409
nutrients, foods, and dietary patterns, 409–411
prevention or treatment of, 406–413
Hypernatremia, dehydration, and hyponatremia, **389–399**
Hyponatremia, bone fractures associated with, 393
causes of, 393–394
definition of, 393

Hyponatremia (*continued*)
delirium and cognitive impairment in, 393
hypernatremia, and dehydration, **389–399**
treatment of, 394
Hypotension, postprandial, 349–350

K

Kidney disease, chronic, protein intake and, 334, 335
Knee arthroplasty, in malnutrition, 334

L

Leucine, anabolic effects of, 332
Lipids, 401
Lipoprotein lipase, 403
Lipoprotein(s), high-density, 403
subclasses, functions, and composition, 402

M

Malnutrition, consequences of, in elderly, 431
hip fracture in, 333–334
knee arthroplasty in, 334
prevalence of, in elderly, 430
risk factors for, in elderly, 431
screening for, in older people, **429–437**
Manometry, to evaluate gastric emptying, 345
Medications, gastric emptying and, 347–350
Muscle mass and strength, protein intake and, 329–330

N

Nutrients, in small intestine, stimulation of phasic pyloric pressure waves and, 346
Nutrition, and cognition, in aging adults, **453–464**
and physical activity, role of, in cholesterol and aging, **401–416**
diabetes, and exercise, **439–451**
effect on cognition, 454
frailty and, 380
Nutrition assessment, mini, 2-step screening process, 433–435
Nutrition assessment tools, Subjective Global Assessment, 432–433
Nutrition-exercise interaction, 446–447
Nutrition screening, 431–435
tools for, 432
Nutritional therapy, in diabetes, 443–444

O

Obesity, detrimental metabolic changes due to, 311–312
in adults, controversy concerning, 313–314
prevalence of, in US, 311, 312

Osteoporosis, protein intake and, 334
vitamin D and, 360

P

Physical activity, and nutrition, role of, in cholesterol and aging, **401–416**
Polyphenols, disease prevention and, 455
Protein, and amino acids, supplementation with, 331–333
and older persons, **327–338**
intake of, amount and timing of, 331–333
and chronic kidney disease, 334, 335
and ideal body weight, 329
and osteoporosis, 334
bone mineral density and, 334
higher, ceiling effect of, on protein synthesis, 333
Protein deficits, age-associated, causes of, 328
intake of, association with muscle mass, muscle strength, and functionality, 329–330
daily, recommendations for, 328–329
in different settings, 329
in older people, 329
consensus recommendations for, 330–331
revelance of, 333–334
Protein requirements, factors affecting, in older age, 327–329
Protein synthesis, effect of higher protein intake on, 333

R

Riboflavin, 361

S

Sarcopenia, and frailty, intervening against, strategies for, 371–372
new conceptual model of, 370–371
studies in parallel, 369–370
as biological substrate of frailty, **367–373**
assessment of, 368–369
definition of, 368
Scintigraphy, to evaluate gastric emptying, 343–344

U

Ultrasonography, to evaluate gastric emptying, 344

V

Vitamin A, and ß-carotene, 356–358
bone health and, 352
cancer prevention and, 357–358
cataracts/macular degeneration and, 358
Vitamin B2, 361

Vitamin B6, 361–362
Vitamin B12, 361–362
Vitamin C (ascorbic acid), 359–360
  cataracts and, 359
  common cold and, 359–360
Vitamin D, 360–361
  and cancer, 360–361
  and diabetes, 361
  cardiovascular disease and, 360
  cognitive function and, 457
  falls and, 360
  osteoporosis and, 360
Vitamin E, 358–359
  cancer prevention and, 358
  cardiovascular disease and, 359
  dementia and, 359
Vitamin requirements, changing over life span, 355
Vitamin status, altered, risk factors for, 356
  medications affecting, 357
Vitamin supplementation, and disease prevention, 356
  in elderly, **355–366**

W

Weight loss, causes of, meals-on-wheels method to screen for, 437
Weight loss interventions, complications and concerns in, 323
  nonpharmacologic, 314–322
Weight loss therapy, clinical outcomes of, 313–323

Printed and bound by CPI Group (UK) Ltd, Croydon, CR0 4YY
03/10/2024
01040490-0015